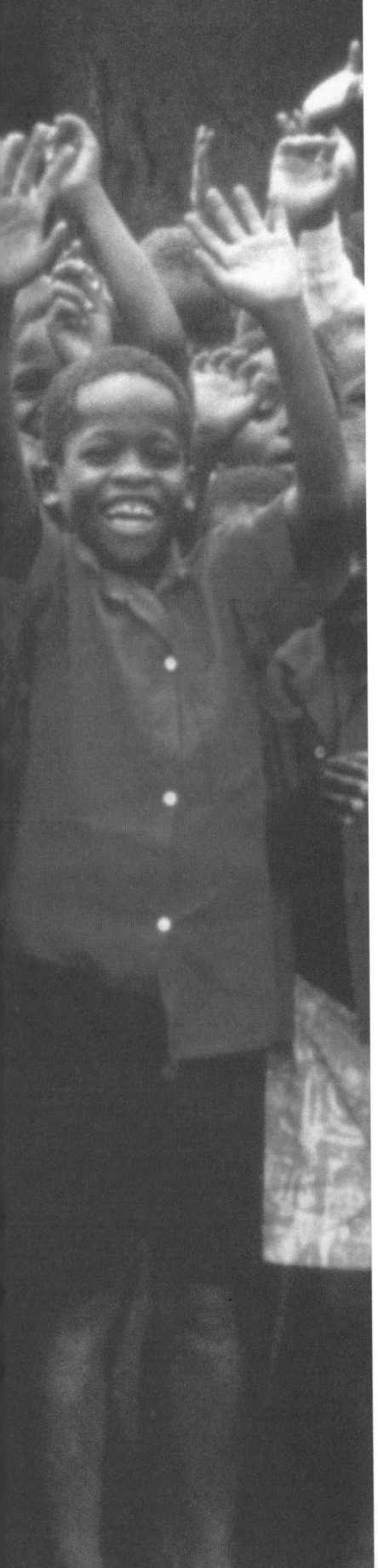
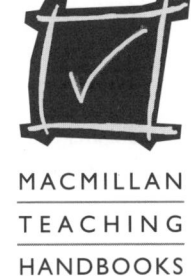

MACMILLAN
TEACHING
HANDBOOKS

Teaching About HIV and AIDS

Maren Bodenstein
Gisela Winkler

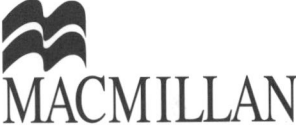

Macmillan Education
4 Crinan Street, London N1 9XW
A division of Macmillan Publishers Limited
Companies and representatives throughout the world

ISBN 978-1-4050-3124-0

Text © Gisela Winkler and Maren Bodenstein 2005
Design and illustration © Macmillan Publishers Limited 2005

First published 2005

All rights reserved; no part of this publication may be reproduced, stored in a retrieval system, transmitted in any form, or by any means, electronic, mechanical, photocopying, recording, or otherwise, without the prior written permission of the publishers.

Typeset by Jim Weaver Design Ltd
Illustrated by Tek Art and Chris Evans
Cover design by Charles Design Associates

The authors and publishers would like to thank Catharine Watson, Uganda; Janet Wildish, CFBT, Kenya; Marianne Christensen, DANIDA, Zambia and Georgina Quaisie, Ghana, for their advice and comments on this text.

The authors and publishers would like to thank the following for permission to reproduce their material:
Straight Talk Foundation for extracts from *Teacher Talk* page 24.
Fr Bernard Joinet for the idea for the illustration on page 50, which is based on the *Fleet of Hope* resources, produced jointly with the Tanzania AIDS project.

The game on page 85 is an adaptation of an original version that appeared in an extract from *Participatory Package and Quality Assurance*, © D Wilson and R Kathuria, Lusaka, Zambia, and published in *Happy, Healthy and Safe: Youth-to-youth learning activities on growing up, relationships, sexual health, HIV/AIDS, life skills*, compiled and edited by Andrew Hobbs et al, Family Health Trust (Anti-AIDS project) Lusaka, Zambia, 1988

The publishers would like to thank Catholic Parochial Primary School for their invaluable support in developing the cover of this book. Cover models are: Mrs Mary O. Amadi, Julie Laval, Joseph Onalo, Elizabeth Ng'ang'a and Timothy Mwangi. Cover photograph by Morris G. M. Keyonzo Photography

Printed and bound in Malaysia

Contents

Preface		v
Introduction		vii

Section 1: What every teacher needs to know about HIV and AIDS

Topic 1	HIV and AIDS in Africa	2
Topic 2	How HIV spreads	4
Topic 3	Universal precautions	8
Topic 4	More information about HIV and AIDS	10
Topic 5	Talking openly about HIV and AIDS	12
Topic 6	Myths and misunderstandings	14
Topic 7	Some cultural practices and social conditions encourage HIV to spread	16
Topic 8	Living positively with HIV	18
Topic 9	Caring for people with AIDS	20
Topic 10	How HIV and AIDS affect our communities and schools	22
Topic 11	Sex and the teacher	24

Section 2: Laying the foundations – understanding our attitudes to HIV and AIDS

Topic 12	What it means to live with HIV and AIDS	26
Topic 13	Helping teachers look at their own risk	28
Topic 14	Understanding our feelings about HIV and AIDS	30
Topic 15	Understanding my own attitudes to HIV and AIDS	32
Topic 16	My community's attitudes towards AIDS	34
Topic 17	Our attitudes towards the children we teach	36

Section 3: Preventing the spread of HIV and AIDS

Topic 18	Education can help prevent the spread of HIV and AIDS	38
Topic 19	What puts children at risk of getting infected with HIV?	40
Topic 20	Sexual abuse	42
Topic 21	Helping young children to stay safe from abuse	44
Topic 22	Changing the way we behave	46
Topic 23	Helping children to make positive choices	48
Topic 24	The ABCD of prevention	50
Topic 25	The A of prevention – Abstaining	52
Topic 26	The B of prevention – Be faithful	56
Topic 27	The C of prevention – Condomise	58
Topic 28	Assertiveness skills	60
Topic 29	Listening skills	62
Topic 30	Resisting peer pressure	64
Topic 31	Starting a Youth HIV and AIDS club	66

Section 4: Sex and sexuality

Topic 32	Our attitudes to sexuality	68
Topic 33	Teaching about sex	70
Topic 34	Teaching about sex at the right level	72
Topic 35	Puberty: the changing body	74
Topic 36	Puberty: the changing personality	76
Topic 37	Dealing with sexual feelings	78
Topic 38	Teaching about sexual intercourse and pregnancy	80

Topic 39	Teaching about HIV and AIDS and other STDs	84
Topic 40	Sex and power	86

Section 5: Teaching about HIV in all areas of the curriculum

Topic 41	When and how to teach about HIV	88
Topic 42	Teaching about HIV and AIDS in all subject areas	90
Topic 43	Using science lessons to teach about HIV and AIDS	92
Topic 44	Using stories and readers to teach about HIV and AIDS	94
Topic 45	Using Social Studies lessons to teach about HIV and AIDS	96
Topic 46	Linking your teaching about HIV and AIDS to life	98
Topic 47	Teaching Life Skills at school	100
Topic 48	Teaching effective communication	102
Topic 49	Nurturing behaviour change	104
Topic 50	Nurturing hope	106

Section 6: Teaching children affected by HIV and AIDS

Topic 51	HIV and AIDS and vulnerable children	108
Topic 52	Understanding vulnerable children	110
Topic 53	Responding to vulnerable children	112
Topic 54	Supporting children with emotional needs	114
Topic 55	Discussing death with children	116
Topic 56	Supporting children in times of grief	118
Topic 57	Teaching large classes	120
Topic 58	Supporting children who are absent from school	122
Topic 59	Creating caring classrooms for children with AIDS	124
Topic 60	The value of home visits	126
Topic 61	Who cares for the carers?	128

Answers to quiz questions throughout book	130
Picture story: A dangerous situation	132
How young people's bodies develop	133

Preface

The HIV and AIDS pandemic stands out as the single most devastating development challenge facing Africa and other continents all over the globe. Two decades since it was first recognised in Africa, the pandemic continues to reverse development gains in the already weak economies of Africa. The spread and impact of HIV and AIDS is cause for global concern because it mainly afflicts young and productive populations in whom the African continent hopes to invest its future. In many of the African countries south of the Sahara, 50 per cent of all new infections with HIV are recognised among young people below the age of 25.

Increasing the access to quality HIV and AIDS information and services for young people has been a major concern among policy-makers and programme planners in Africa, as well as among education authorities, currently implementing a multi-sectoral response to the pandemic.

Many factors increase the risk of young people being infected with HIV: they include socio-cultural, socio-economic, psycho-social and emotional circumstances, all of which vary in degree from one community to another.

In most parts of Africa, poverty levels are high, while school enrolment is low and there is a poor record of primary school completion. This leads to most young people, especially girls, remaining subject to traditional values and norms, such as early marriages, sex for favours and other traditional practices that increase the risk of infection. Unfortunately, due to cultural inhibitions and other factors, most parents find it difficult to talk about sexuality with their children. As a result, they are not given basic facts about how HIV is transmitted and what precautions they should take. Moreover, the age of onset of sexual activity in some African countries is as low as 13 years, with girls being reported to be five times higher at risk of HIV infection than their male counterparts.

The general lack of openness about HIV and AIDS makes it difficult to dispel the many myths and misconceptions that young people pick up from their peers, and this reduces prevention opportunities. The problem is compounded by the increasing number of children being made orphans and, therefore, vulnerable as a result of the impact of HIV and AIDS. Additionally, many are being turned into care-givers by their sick and ailing parents, thus depriving them of the opportunity to remain in school, despite the major efforts currently being made in Africa to increase the success of universal primary education (UPE).

The need to intensify AIDS education in schools has become more urgent with the increasing demands placed on the teachers as UPE takes root and more children enrol in schools. Many parents spend less and less time with their children, and do not give the necessary guidance to impart skills that would enable their children to protect themselves from infection. To overcome this problem, the capacity of teachers to teach about HIV and AIDS must be strengthened through the mainstreaming of HIV and AIDS in the teacher-training curriculum; an infusion of the AIDS content in the in-service and other continuing education programmes for teachers; regular support, monitoring, supervision and the provision of relevant materials.

Teaching about AIDS in schools is bound to meet certain challenges, especially in Africa, where attitudes, beliefs and practices handed down from one generation to another, have a lot of influence in adulthood. It is therefore inevitable that the teachers' own attitudes and their personal perception of risk, will be heavily influenced by their community's attitude towards HIV and AIDS. This may have a negative effect on the manner in which they teach their children about the subject.

But teachers are change agents in their schools and in their local communities and many are so highly valued in the localities where they teach that their opinion is sought for every new development programme. Even political leaders rely on teachers to influence or swing voting patterns during electioneering campaigns in rural areas.

Engaging teachers, their employers (e.g. Teachers Service Commissions) and their trade unions in the fight against HIV and AIDS in a constructive and participatory manner will be of enormous help in the

Teaching about HIV and AIDS

war against HIV and AIDS among young people. Teachers have the potential to influence and inculcate the values and virtues of self control, assertiveness and other life skills that young people need to enable them cope with the challenges of the pandemic. In addition, teachers can facilitate the cascading and uptake of proven interventions. For example, they can encourage abstinence and help children to make informed choices.

It is, therefore, critical for teachers to be thoroughly equipped with knowledge about HIV and AIDS, to be aware of all the issues around the disease and be adequately empowered to teach the subject in many different circumstances. Importantly, they must be able to adapt their teaching to the needs and cultural orientations of young people from various backgrounds.

This book is intended for student teachers, teachers and guidance/counselling staff in schools, as well as education sector policy-makers and programme-planners. It covers a wide spectrum of HIV/AIDS as a core subject in schools and provides a variety of approaches and options for teaching the subject. Although it will be especially useful to teachers in developing countries, it could also benefit those in the developed world.

In my work on HIV and AIDS, which has spanned more than 12 years, I have laid great emphasis on working with young people as the priority intervention to reverse the rising tide of the pandemic in our hard-hit countries. Young people are the future of every society, and protecting them from this deadly scourge guarantees continuity of human capital for the development of any nation. Teachers have a central role in shaping the future of young people at every level of education and should be encouraged not only to teach the subject, but to strive to be role models.

I strongly recommend this comprehensive, thoroughly-researched and well-presented, easy-to-read book to all involved in educating primary school children: pre-service and in-service primary teacher educators, co-ordinators and managers of teacher advisory resource centres, primary school heads, student teachers on teaching practice or in colleges, primary school inspectors and, of course, serving primary school teachers.

Dr Meshack H O Ndolo, MPH
Deputy Programme Manager, Kenya National AIDS/STD Control Programme
and HIV/AIDS and Development Consultant

Introduction

Macmillan Teaching Handbooks

This series has been designed for student and practising primary teachers in African schools and teacher training colleges. It has been developed as a result of consultation with practising teachers, student teachers and college teacher trainers. The series includes this book, *Teaching About HIV and AIDS*, one on Primary Teaching Methods, one each for the main subjects: English, Science, Mathematics, and Social Studies, and one for Reading. All books cover upper and lower primary.

The books are designed to be used by unqualified or newly-qualified teachers, by students studying on formal college courses and by experienced teachers who wish to improve their practice. Readers are encouraged to try out methods and strategies to improve learning and to reflect on their own teaching, either individually or in groups. The material can also be used in Teacher Training College courses or, equally effectively, in school-based staff development programmes supported by the headteacher, teachers themselves or by primary school advisors.

The books present the material in an attractive, easy-to-use form, without compromising on concept level, coverage or depth. They make no assumptions about previous study or knowledge, they avoid jargon and use clear language. They provide a wealth of practical suggestions and ideas, keeping in mind the problems and challenges that teachers face in the classroom.

Teaching About HIV and AIDS

This area of the curriculum is a challenging one to teach, for many reasons. This book covers all that the aspiring or busy teacher needs to know to begin teaching about HIV and AIDS. It provides clear, accurate information for the teacher, along with activities to encourage reflection and better practice, and suggestions for how to tackle the various aspects of HIV and AIDS education and difficult issues in the classroom. It also includes advice and suggestions to help teachers and children affected by HIV and AIDS.

The book has six sections: *1 What every teacher needs to know about HIV and AIDS*; *2 Laying the foundations – understanding our attitudes to HIV and AIDS*; *3 Preventing the spread of HIV and AIDS*; *4 Sex and sexuality*; *5 Teaching about HIV in all areas of the curriculum*; *6 Teaching children affected by HIV and AIDS*.

Each section is divided into a number of topics. The sections and topics have been grouped in a particular order to lead readers through important ideas and issues, but the book does not have to be read through from the beginning. Readers may have different priorities and each topic, while designed to stand alone, has been linked to others by cross-referencing. This means that readers can quickly and easily refer to particular topics and linked themes.

Each topic covers either one or two double-page spreads, containing background information and classroom ideas to encourage readers to try out new ideas. They include simple definitions of terms and examples of approaches that other teachers have found effective. All topics contain activities to help teachers develop as professionals. These encourage readers to:
- assess their own knowledge and skills;
- understand their own attitudes to HIV and AIDS and those of their pupils;
- develop a variety of teaching methods and strategies that will improve their pupils' learning;
- create caring classrooms, where HIV and AIDS can be discussed openly.

This book contains information about HIV and AIDS and sex education, which some readers will find sensitive. Teachers need to be fully and accurately informed about HIV and AIDS in order to teach effectively and take their part in preventing the spread of the disease. But please remember that this book

Teaching about HIV and AIDS

is for teachers and **not for pupils**. Teachers need to use their professional expertise in order to decide exactly what level and kind of knowledge to teach their pupils. This expertise will be related to their school policies and teachers will bear in mind their knowledge of the children they teach and the communities in which they serve. We must also keep in mind the fact that many children leave school after primary education, so primary children need to know the information that will keep them safe in later life.

It is also important to remember that it is a teacher's duty to teach accurately, and in a way which keeps the children as safe as possible. Some people oppose providing information to young people about sex because they think it will encourage them to experiment and take more risks. Researchers from international organisations such as the World Health Organisation and UNAIDS have carefully studied the effects of sex education programmes and have found that the results are exactly the opposite. Providing accurate and honest information about sex encourages young people to delay having sex and take action to protect themselves.

Teaching About HIV and AIDS

Section 1 What every teacher needs to know about HIV and AIDS

1 HIV and AIDS in Africa

Definitions

HIV stands for Human Immunodeficiency Virus.

AIDS stands for Acquired Immune Deficiency Syndrome.

An **epidemic** is a disease that spreads quickly and cannot easily be controlled.

Did you know?

The time that passes between HIV infection and the first signs of AIDS will be different for every person and it is difficult to predict how well the body can defend itself against HIV.

- Some people are **rapid progressors**. This means they will quickly develop severe illnesses and could die within two or three years of becoming infected with HIV.
- Most people are **slow progressors**. They can live between five and eight years before they have AIDS.
- A few people are **long-term survivors**. They live for many years with HIV before they become seriously ill. A very few people have HIV but do not become sick.

The immune system

We all have a system in our body that fights off infections and diseases. It is called **the immune system**. HIV is a virus that slowly breaks down our immune system. At first, this does not seem like a big problem at all. A person with HIV can look good and feel well for quite a long time. As time passes, the immune system of a person with HIV will become weaker and the body is no longer able to fight off infections. When the virus has permanently damaged the immune system, HIV turns into AIDS. A person with AIDS becomes ill very often and also takes a long time to recover from each illness.

How HIV progresses to AIDS

Phase 1 is the point of infection, when HIV enters a living human body. A person can be infected several times over.

Phase 2 is the invisible disease, which lasts up to eight years, or even longer. During this time, HIV lives and multiplies in the body. The person living with HIV is able to infect others without knowing. Continued exposure to sexual risk can shorten Phase 2, but there are behaviours which extend life expectancy (eating nutritious food, avoiding stresses such as alcohol, treating all illnesses quickly with prescribed medical treatment, testing for and treating TB).

Phase 3 is the visible disease – AIDS. Antiretroviral drugs (ARVs) can often be used effectively at this stage and are usually only given when the immune system is already very weak. (See Topic 4, page 10, and Topic 8, page 19).

How can we tell if we have HIV?

It is important to think about the time-gap between HIV infections and first signs of AIDS. During this period, there are no outward signs that can tell us if we are living with HIV or not. Unless we take a blood test for HIV, we will not know if we have the virus and if we are passing it on. This means it is impossible to 'see' the HIV problem or to know how fast HIV is spreading in our communities. HIV is invisible for a long time, and this makes it very difficult to protect

From HIV to AIDS

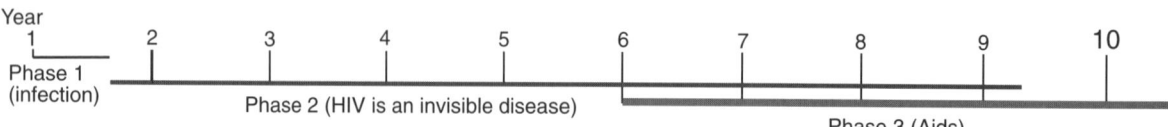

A typical timeline between infection with HIV and the onset of AIDS.

What every teacher needs to know about HIV and AIDS

> **Activity** Finish this paragraph
>
> How would you finish this paragraph on HIV and AIDS in Africa? Reflect on your own experience to help you.
>
> *'HIV is a virus that has been around since the late 1970s. Although many people have made an effort to stop the virus, it has spread quickly across Africa. HIV has become an epidemic and we are still without a cure. In all these years, life in our communities went on. Parents with HIV sent their children to school. Teachers with HIV went on teaching, and children with HIV went on trying to learn. But then things began to change. HIV infections started to turn into AIDS ...*
> *..................................,'*

> *A possible response*
>
> Now that people have seen the devastation caused by HIV they are trying to protect their communities by sharing their knowledge about the disease, encouraging people to avoid behaviour that increases the risk of infection and looking at how the community can support individuals in this change.

young people from becoming infected with the disease. They believe that the healthy-looking person in front of them cannot be infected.

Many people only begin to understand that HIV is a problem when their friends and family begin to die of AIDS. They notice that HIV is affecting their community when people become poorer, because they are too ill to work. Others notice that children leave school to care for their families or to find work.

Ideas for the classroom

Before you start teaching about HIV and AIDS, it is important to listen to the children and find out what they already know about the disease. What do they understand? What do they misunderstand?

Question the children about what they know. Challenge any misconceptions (such as, that everyone with HIV will die soon and that HIV and AIDS are the same thing) and guide the discussion. Your questions will depend on what you want the children to learn. For example, do you want them to increase their knowledge about risk, or to reduce stigma?

Following this, ask the children to draw constructive pictures about HIV and AIDS, such as caring for someone who is sick or showing how to prevent HIV.

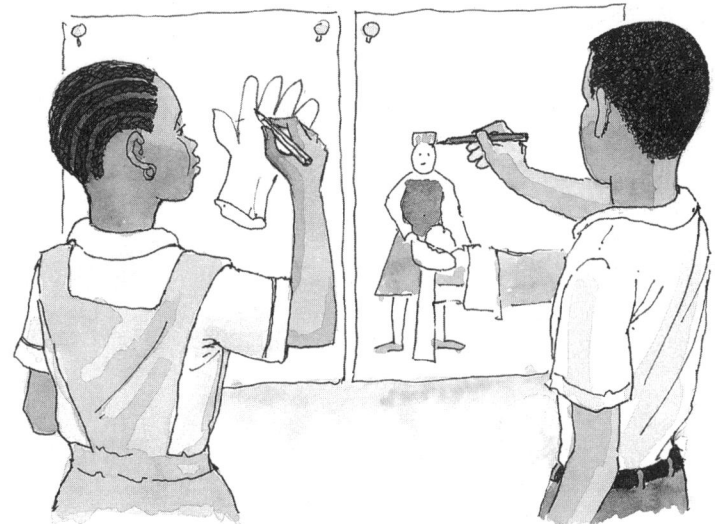

> *Helpful hints*
>
> These questions can help you to think about the pictures children draw.
> - Do the children see a difference between HIV and AIDS?
> - What ideas about HIV and AIDS are most common?
> - Where do their ideas about HIV come from? The curriculum? The media? Personal experience?
> - Which images present incorrect information about HIV and AIDS? How can you correct this?

2 How HIV spreads

Definitions

Body fluids include blood, semen and vaginal fluids. These can carry HIV. Others body fluids, such as urine, vomit and faeces, do not in themselves carry HIV. But they can do so when they contain blood.

The **window period** is the time after the HIV infection, when the virus is in the body, but does not yet show up in a blood test.

HIV antibodies are special cells the body makes in response to becoming infected with HIV. The job of HIV antibodies is to fight the HIV infection.

What HIV needs to spread

HIV is a virus that lives in our body cells and is present in some body fluids. Blood, semen (the fluid that carries the male's sperm) and vaginal fluid can contain HIV. HIV can only be passed on from one person to another, when the body fluids of an infected person enter another person's body. There needs to be:

1 A route of exit from one body, e.g. a bleeding wound or sexual ejaculation.
2 An entry point into another person's body, e.g. a cut in the skin. Entry points can include a bruise or micro-lacerations (tiny cuts in the skin, which cannot be seen and which are most likely in soft tissue, such as inside the vagina and on the surface of the penis).

When HIV spreads

HIV can spread when:

- people have sex;
- women are pregnant, give birth or are breastfeeding (HIV is spread from mother to baby);
- blood containing HIV goes from one person and enters another.

There is no risk of getting HIV when there is no contact with body fluids.

HIV is **not spread** by:

- touching
- holding hands
- hugging or by kissing (unless the person has open sores in their mouth).

It is also **not spread by** sharing cups and plates, sharing toilets or giving blood using sterilised equipment.

Sexual transmission

For the most part, HIV is a sexually transmitted disease. The virus will be in the semen (the liquid that carries the male sperm) or the vaginal fluids of the person who is infected with HIV. When people have unprotected sex, the virus can easily pass from one body to the next.

The risk of HIV infection during sex is even higher if one of the partners has a sexually transmitted disease, such as genital herpes, gonorrhoea or syphilis.

Mother-to-child transmission

HIV can also pass from mother to baby. This can happen when the mother is carrying the baby in her womb and during delivery, when the new-born baby is in contact with the mother's blood and vaginal fluids. Transmission can also happen through breastfeeding.

What every teacher needs to know about HIV and AIDS

How HIV spreads

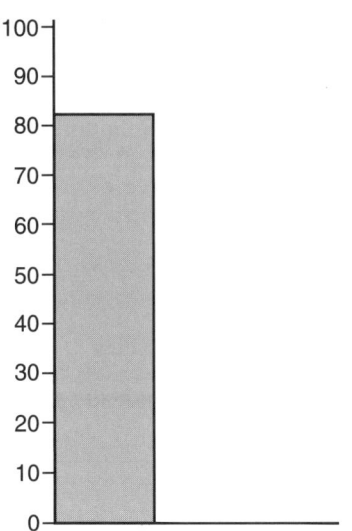

Through sex: over 80 per cent of all people living with HIV in Africa got infected through sex.

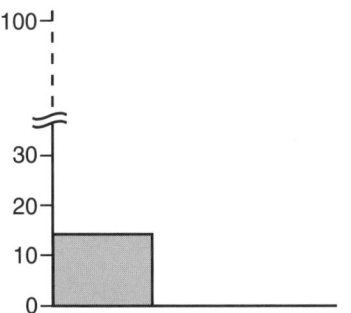

Mother-to-child: About 14 per cent of people living with HIV in Africa were infected this way.

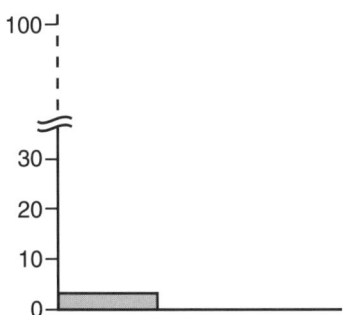

Blood: Two per cent of people living with HIV in Africa were infected this way.

Blood and blood products

HIV can be passed on by infected blood – from unsterilised needles used for injections, or blood transfusions that have not been checked properly, or when blood from an infected person flows into an open cut on someone else. This means it can be passed on when people with HIV are injured and bleed onto one another, or when they share needles for injecting medicines and drugs, or when small amounts of blood are transferred from one infected person into another person through or by a shared razor, needle or earring.

> *Did you know?*
>
> The most commonly used HIV tests are not looking for the actual virus that makes someone HIV positive. They measure HIV antibodies in the blood or saliva. The HIV antibodies are special cells made by the body to fight the HIV infection.

The window period

If a person is infected with HIV, it takes a few weeks before HIV antibodies show up in an HIV test. This means there is a time when the virus is in the body, but cannot yet be traced. This time is called the **window period**. The window period lasts about three months. Some doctors advise people to have an HIV test twice, separated by three to four months, to make sure the window period is over and the result of the test is accurate.

Activity Thinking about sex education

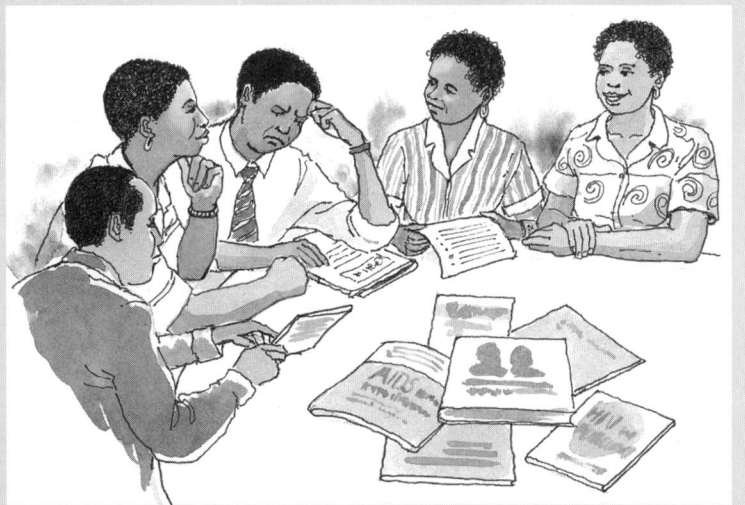

Having sex is the most common way in which people get HIV. This is true for adults, and also for children who are still at school. How do you see the role of sex education in the fight against HIV and AIDS? Discuss this with your colleagues.

Teaching about HIV and AIDS

Activity

Plan a lesson on *How to stay safe*. Clearly state the age of the children you have in mind. Make sure your lesson is at the right level for this age. Include an exercise that helps children see the importance of abstaining or delaying sex.

Did you know?

There are drugs to reduce the risk of mother-to-child transmission of HIV. When a woman with HIV uses these drugs during her pregnancy the child has a good chance of being born without HIV. That is why many hospitals encourage pregnant women to test for HIV and to take the treatment as prescribed.

How to stay safe

- **If you are a virgin**

Delay starting sex: do not have sex and do not allow anyone to have sex with you. Ideally, abstain until marriage or until you have a partner for life.

- **If you have already had sex**

Make a decision to stop until you are married or have a partner for life. Before you have sex for the first time, take an HIV test with your partner.

- **If you are married**

Be faithful to your uninfected partner. Do not assume your partner is faithful, so talk about your relationship and staying safe together. Use condoms, unless you want to have a child.

- **If you are a sexually active adult with more than one partner**

Take an HIV test to find out your status. Always use condoms correctly every time you have sex. Do not have casual sex. Try to reduce the number of partners you have. Talk about how to stay safe with your sexual partners.

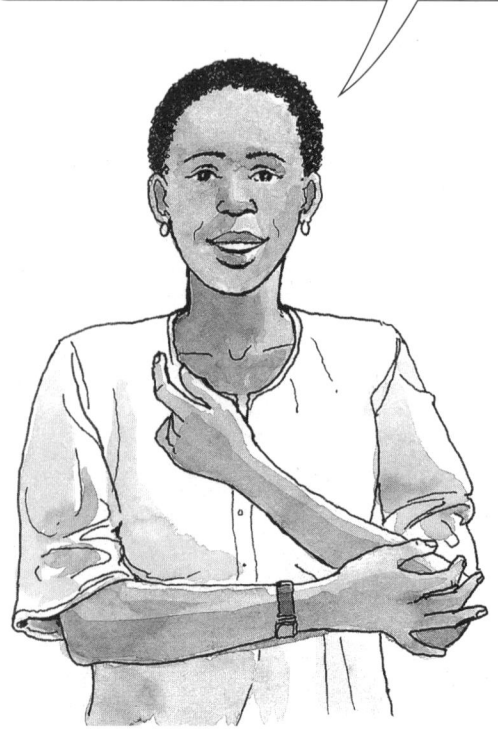

I used to be afraid of HIV and AIDS. What if my neighbour has it and I don't know? Then I found out that I can only get infected if I have unsafe sex with a person who has HIV, or if his blood passes into mine. Now I know how to judge the risk of getting HIV. For women like me, there are many situations that can be risky, because there is a lot of sexual violence in our community. It is hard to deny a man when he wants sex. For the sake of our children these attitudes must change. I believe we must teach our children, especially our girls, to notice when a situation is risky, and to get out. We must teach them to keep themselves safe.

What every teacher needs to know about HIV and AIDS

Activity   Keeping children safe

When are children in your community at risk of being forced into sex?
Make a list of the 'high risk' situations you worry about.
What information, skills and support from adults do children need to stay safe?

Activity

Plan a lesson to teach children about the ways HIV is transmitted and how it cannot be spread. Make a list of those things which are safe: e.g., hugging or sharing plates with people who have HIV. State clearly the age of the children the lesson is designed for.

Helpful hints

- Be clear and open about the way HIV is spread. If a child asks how HIV is spread, tell them the three ways outlined on these pages and explain that the virus needs an exit from one person and an entry to the second person.
- Show acceptance of people living with HIV.
- Allow time for questions and discussions. Allow pupils to discuss in pairs or groups and feed back to the class.
- Remember that teaching a child to listen to their inner voice about feeling safe and unsafe is an important life skill. (See also Topic 21, page 44, *Helping young children to stay safe from abuse*.)

Ideas for the classroom

Here is a lesson that helps you to check if children understand how HIV spreads.

Tell the children to close their eyes and cross their hands in front of their chests.

Then ask them to listen to a statement you will read out.

If they agree with the statement, they must stretch their hands up to the sky.

If they disagree with the statement, they must point their hands to the floor.

Only when all the children have decided on their answer are they allowed to open their eyes and look around.

As a teacher, you can then talk about the statement with the class.

At the end of each round, repeat the statement and give the correct answer.

Here are some examples of statements you can read to the class.

- You can get HIV from toilet seats.
  (Answer: disagree. However, it is good to keep toilets clean, so no germs can spread.)
- A pregnant mother with HIV will ALWAYS infect her baby.
  (Answer: disagree. There is a 50 per cent chance that the mother will pass the virus on to the baby. There are drugs available to reduce the risk of transmission even further. See page 6, opposite.)
- If you have sex you are at risk of getting HIV.
  (Answer: agree. Sex is the most common way in which HIV is transmitted.)
- If you have sex with only one person, you will not get HIV.
  (Answer: disagree. If the one person you have sex with is infected with HIV, you can get HIV from him or her.)

3 Universal precautions

Definition

Universal precautions mean we make sure we have no direct contact with any body fluids that could contain HIV. **These precautions are universal because they are applied to all people, in all situations and to all body fluids.**

Protecting ourselves

One important way in which we can protect ourselves from the spread of HIV and other infections is to practise **universal precautions**.

When we take universal precautions we make sure we do not touch any body fluids of any person at any time. That way we avoid the risk of getting infections. It does not matter if a person has HIV or not. Universal precautions are helpful because they keep everybody safe and do not discriminate against people with HIV. Teaching children about universal precautions can be a good way of teaching children about HIV without blaming anyone for the disease.

Universal precautions for teachers

- Keep a First Aid Kit close at hand (see Activity).
- Teach children to stop their own bleeding by taking a clean cloth or paper and pressing hard. Sometimes children prefer to suck their skin if it bleeds, and this is OK.
- Teach children not to touch other people's blood.
- Use gloves or plastic bags to cover your hands when helping children who are injured or sick.
- Stop all bleeding as quickly as possible.
- Clean the wounds by patting them gently with a clean cloth or cotton wool dipped in antiseptic.
- Use antiseptic or diluted bleach to clean all areas that have come into contact with vomit, diarrhoea or blood.
- Make arrangements to dispose of sanitary towels or tampons at the school, so no one can have contact with them.

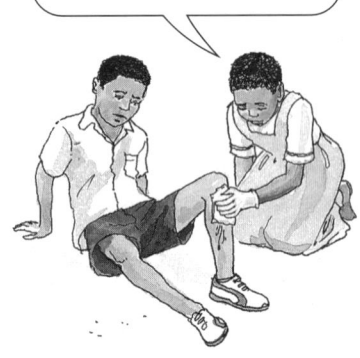

That hurts! Here, press hard. That will stop the bleeding. I'll call the teacher to help you clean the wound.

Activity Make your own First Aid kit for the playground

Make sure your First Aid kit is in a small bag that you can easily carry with you when you are on duty outside.

Your bag should contain a pair of plastic gloves (rubber household gloves will do), a small bottle of antiseptic fluid, some cotton wool, some clean pieces of cloth, a bandage, a plastic bag for soiled and bloody material.

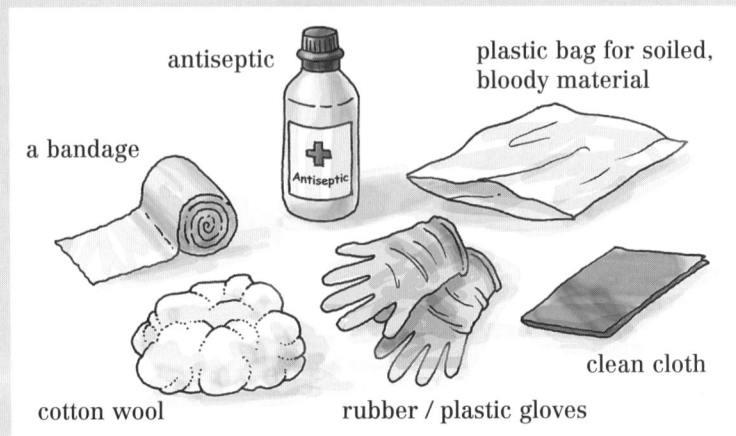

What every teacher needs to know about HIV and AIDS

Remember

You can dilute ordinary household bleach to clean wounds. Usually you mix one part of bleach with five parts of water. However, since concentrations of bleach may vary, you should always read the instructions on the bottle. If you use a bleach solution to sterilise instruments, keep the instruments in the mixture for at least 30 minutes.

Did you know?

Keeping healthy

People with AIDS become ill easily, as their immune systems no longer work well. A person with a healthy immune system can fight germs much more easily. Where a healthy child will only get a cold, a child suffering from AIDS might get pneumonia or even die. If we are living in a community where people are suffering from AIDS, it is very important to teach children the basic rules of hygiene to keep one another safe. Remind them:

- to wash their hands before they eat
- to wash their hands after they have used a toilet
- to cover their faces when they sneeze or cough
- always to sleep under a mosquito net if they live in an area where there is malaria
- not to spit.

Helpful hints

- **Be kind and show empathy**

Talk about universal precautions in a calm and open way. It does not help to scare children with the threat of HIV. Even in a community without HIV, universal precautions are an important life skill.

- **Be practical**

Make sure the children have a chance to practise putting on gloves or using plastic bags and clean imaginary wounds. Universal precautions need both knowledge and skill. You will get into the habit if you practise them all the time.

Ideas for the classroom

Tell your class about universal precautions and why they are important.

Divide the class into groups and ask each group to prepare a short radio song to advertise universal precautions. Encourage the groups to find creative ways to make the message stick.

Each group then presents the advertisements to the class.

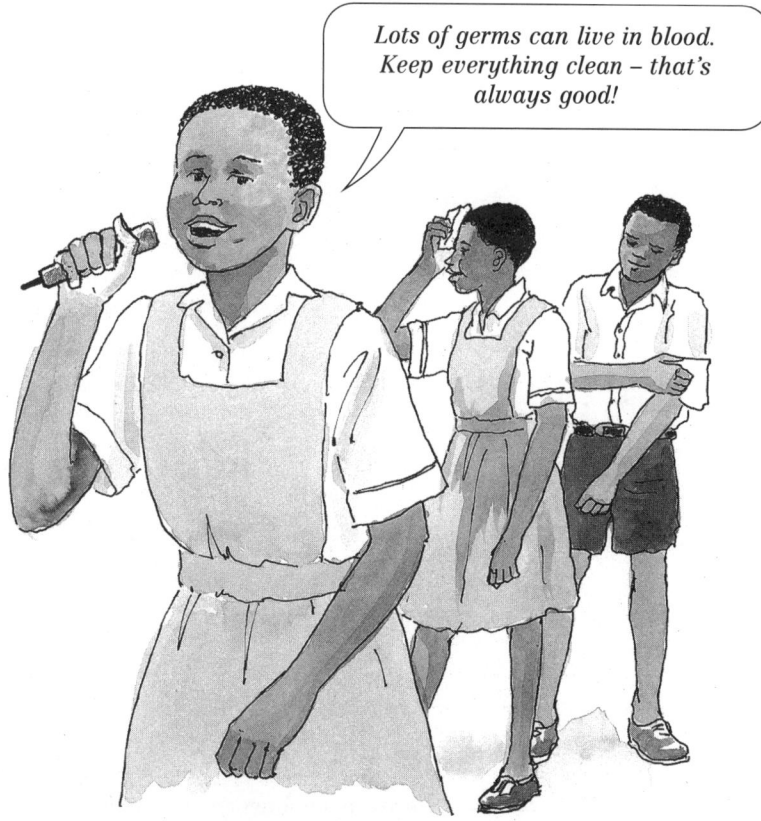

4 More information about HIV and AIDS

Definitions

T-cells are special blood cells that fight infections.

CD4 cells are special T-cells that tell other T-cells what to do. Without CD4 cells, our bodies have no protection against infections and diseases.

Antiretroviral drugs can stop HIV attacking and growing inside CD4 cells, but this does not last for ever.

The nucleus is the central part of a cell.

HIV and the immune system

The immune system of the human body uses white blood cells to defend itself against germs. Some of the white blood cells are called T-cells. T-cells are 'fighter cells' that protect the body from infections.

CD4 cells are a special kind of T-cells, also called T4 lymphocytes, which tell other fighter cells what to do. Without CD4 cells, the other cells will not know how to fight diseases. When HIV gets into the body, it attacks the CD4 cells. The following diagram shows you how this attack works.

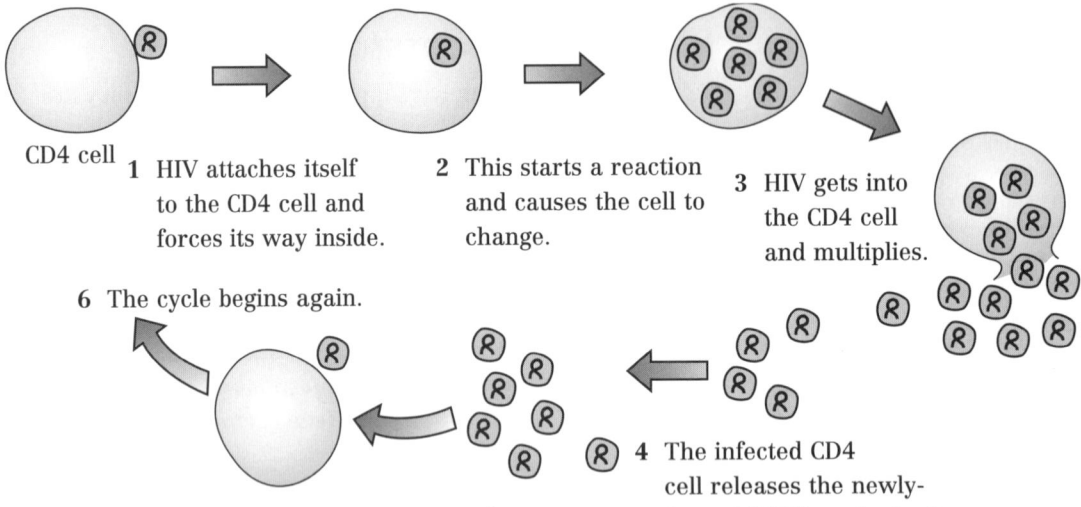

CD4 cell
1 HIV attaches itself to the CD4 cell and forces its way inside.
2 This starts a reaction and causes the cell to change.
3 HIV gets into the CD4 cell and multiplies.
4 The infected CD4 cell releases the newly-formed HIV into the body.
5 The new viruses spread out, ready to attack other CD4 cells.
6 The cycle begins again.

Did you know?

Scientists from all over the world have been studying HIV for many years. They have not yet found a cure for AIDS. But they have developed drugs to help people living with HIV. These are called **antiretroviral drugs** (or ARVs) and they attack HIV in the body. ARVs make it difficult for the virus to multiply and spread. These drugs cannot cure the HIV infection, but they can help people who are infected to live longer and healthier lives.

Activity Evaluate your own understanding about HIV and AIDS

1 What is the difference between HIV and AIDS?
2 When HIV enters the body there is a 'window period' during which an HIV test will not show infection, because the test looks for antibodies that have not yet been made. Which part of the above diagram shows the window period?
3 Why are T-cells important?

(You can find the answers to these questions on this page and on page 130.)

Getting AIDS

There comes a time when HIV has attacked and changed so many T-cells in the body that it can no longer fight off infections. Then people living with HIV start to show signs of AIDS. AIDS is a combination of illnesses, which tell us that the immune system is no longer doing its job.

What every teacher needs to know about HIV and AIDS

Stage 1: First signs of HIV related infections
Swollen glands
Sweating at night
Mouth ulcers
Oral thrush
Shingles
Fungal infections
Loss of weight (more than 10 per cent of normal body weight)

Stage 2: Major signs of HIV-related infections
Persistent fever (longer than a month)
Severe tiredness
Persistent diarrhoea (longer than a month)
Persistent coughing
Persistent skin rashes and shingles (*herpes zoster*)
Loss of weight (more than 10 per cent of normal body weight)

Stage 3: AIDS
Persistent fever
Persistent diarrhoea
Kaposi's Sarcoma (a cancer-like growth of the blood vessels that can be seen on the skin)
Meningitis
Pneumonia

Signs and symptoms

All the signs or symptoms of HIV/AIDS can also be present because of other diseases, many of which can be cured. A person with any of these symptoms should consult a doctor or health worker to get treatment. **Remember, HIV can only be diagnosed through a blood test. A person with any or all of the symptoms in the diagram above may not necessarily have HIV.**

Helpful hints for the drama

- Make sure all the children understand the process of infection so they know what to do during the drama exercise.
- Work in an open space like a hall, or outside. You could draw a big shape of the body on the floor with chalk or scratch it in the sand.
- Allow children to dress up, so it is easier to see who is who. Examples: let all T-cells wear a cap or hat, give all viruses a red ribbon or cloth.

(See Topic 8, page 18, *Living Positively with HIV* for information about treating HIV with ARVs.)

Ideas for the classroom

Plan a drama exercise for children on how HIV attacks the immune system. Use the information in the diagram on the page opposite to teach the children what to do. Some children will form circles to make up CD4 cells, while other children will pretend to be HIV. Some children can be ARVs that help T-cells fight off HIV.

To make sure the exercise does not become too chaotic, announce each step, before the children move. You can say things like, 'When HIV enters the body the T-cells try to fight off the virus. But in the end some HIV cells get to the CD-4 cells and force their way inside.'

Then give the children a chance to act this part. When you ring a bell or clap your hands, they freeze and you explain the next step.

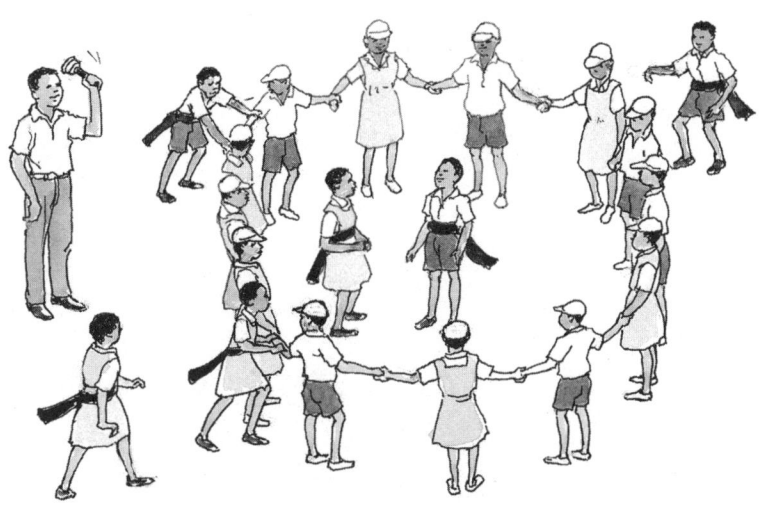

Activity List your questions about the signs of AIDS
- Do you have any questions about how to care for people suffering from AIDS?
- Who can help you answer these questions? Discuss these questions with your colleagues.

5 Talking openly about HIV and AIDS

> **Definition**
>
> A **case study** is a short report about a real-life situation. It usually tells you how one person responds to a particular problem.

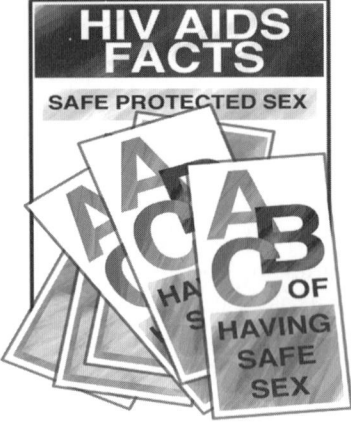

There are many sources of information about sex and HIV.

You cannot teach children about HIV and AIDS without talking openly about sex.

Overcoming your own difficulties

For many adults, talking about sex is a difficult thing to do. As a result, they use unclear language and hint at a situation, saying things like 'you know what I mean'. Even if children hear a lot about HIV and AIDS, not all the information they get is accurate and clear. When people are too shy to speak openly about sexual matters, it does not take long for myths and misunderstandings about the disease to spread.

Will talking about sexuality affect my reputation?

Shyness and ignorance are only two reasons why it is difficult to speak openly about sex and HIV. The third reason has to do with a teacher's feelings of self-respect. Sometimes teachers have all the correct information, but they worry that talking about sexuality will ruin their reputation. They keep quiet, even if they have valuable insights to share.

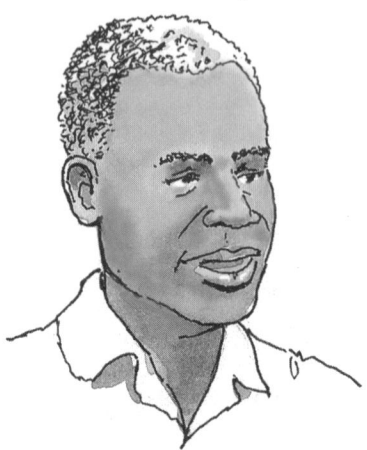

> **Case study**
>
> A teacher from Zambia writes:
>
> I am very worried about the spread of HIV in our community and so I have read a lot about the way the virus spreads. I know that sex education is very important if we want to stop the disease and I have done a course to help me teach about sex and HIV. But I still have problems feeling free in the way I speak. If I explain to my pupils about condoms, for example, they think I know about them because I am sleeping around. That makes me feel very uncomfortable. But if I tell them I learnt about condoms on a course they will laugh at me. They will think I do not really know what is going on. Whichever way I look at it, teaching about sexuality can undermine my position of authority. What should I do?

> **Activity** Thinking about the case study
>
> How does the letter from the teacher in Zambia make you feel?
>
> What advice would you give this teacher?

What every teacher needs to know about HIV and AIDS

Activity *Evaluate yourself*
- How sure are you about your facts? Is there anything you are unsure about?
- From where do you get your information about sex? Is it a reliable source?

As teachers we often teach about things we have not experienced ourselves. Why is personal experience and personal reputation so closely linked to teaching about sexuality and HIV?

Did you know?

When you teach about sex and HIV and AIDS your authority comes from inside you and does not depend on what others think. Your authority is rooted in:
- having accurate information about sexuality and its link with HIV
- your caring about the health and safety of your pupils
- your commitment to compassionate and respectful human relationships
- your personal confidence and attitude to your work.

Ideas for the classroom

Have a question box in your classroom. Encourage the children in your class to write down any questions they have about HIV, AIDS or sex education issues on a piece of paper and put their questions in the box. Tell them to write their questions anonymously (not to put their names on them). Tell them that you (or a health worker, if you prefer) will answer the questions truthfully. Make sure that, even if you recognise the handwriting, you do not give away who has asked which question.

Have a time each week for answering the questions. Do this in a clear, truthful, accurate and friendly way. Leave the box in a corner of the room so that pupils can put in questions without being seen. To begin with you might tell all the pupils that they must each think of a question to put in – then you can answer those and any additional ones over the first few weeks.

Helpful hints
- Sometimes, it is easier to talk about sex when boys and girls attend separate classes.
- Strengthen your position of authority by making clear rules that make it easier for everyone to speak openly about sexual matters. Below are some helpful rules.

1. We respect our bodies and do not laugh and tease about sexual matters.
2. If you are too shy to ask a question, write it on a piece of paper and put it in the question box.
3. All honest questions deserve honest answers.

(The next page gives more information about myths and how to deal with them.)

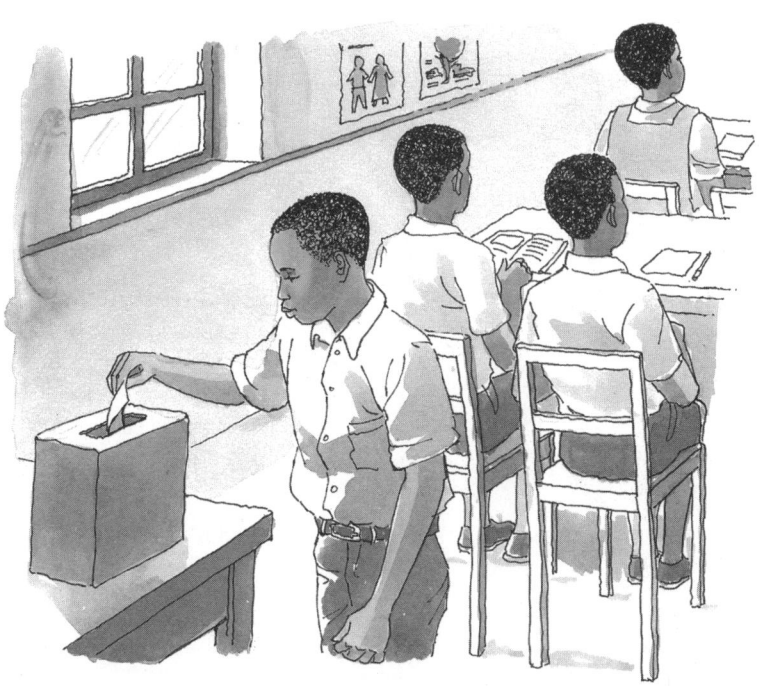

6 Myths and misunderstandings

> ### Definition
> **A myth** is something many people believe, but which is not true.
>
> Typical myths about HIV and AIDS include:
> Sex with a virgin will cure AIDS. ✗
> Witchcraft causes AIDS. ✗
> HIV can pass through condoms. ✗

Knowing what to believe

Although there is a lot of information available about HIV and AIDS, it is not always easy to know what to believe. It is a complex subject and some information is changing as more scientific research is done. Some information available is biased or presents a particular emphasis or moral view.

When you read or hear information about HIV and AIDS, ask yourself where it comes from. Is it a reliable source? If children say things you know to be incorrect, make sure you challenge them and give the correct information instead.

> ### Some facts that pupils need to know
> If you are teaching about HIV/AIDS, there are some important things your pupils need to know.
>
> - Withdrawal just before ejaculation **does not** prevent HIV and AIDS. ✔
> - Washing private parts with disinfectant soon after sex **does not** wash away the virus. ✔
> - A circumcised person can also catch the virus easily. ✔
> - Sex with virgins **does not** cure AIDS. ✔
> - Sex with young children **does not** stop one from getting HIV or AIDS. ✔
> - Having sex with people with disabilities **does not** stop you from getting AIDS. ✔
> - Traditional medicine **does not** cure AIDS. ✔
> - Witchcraft **does not** cause AIDS. ✔
>
> There are also a lot of **false** beliefs about sex that make young people vulnerable to HIV. Help your pupils to be critical of sentences like those following.
> - If you do not have sex, you will go mad. ✗
> - You need to have sex to grow breasts and buttocks. ✗
> - If you do not have sex, your private parts will shrivel up. ✗
> - Boys cannot control their sexual urges. ✗
> - Girls say 'No' but they often really mean 'Yes'. ✗
>
> Be aware of these **myths about condoms**.
> - Condoms have HIV or other germs inside. ✗
> - A bent penis will not fit into a condom. ✗
> - Condoms get stuck inside a woman's body. ✗
> - Condoms cause cancer. ✗
> - You don't have to use a condom every time. ✗
> - Condoms have small holes through which the virus can pass. ✗
>
> (See also Topic 27, page 58.)

Activity Evaluate yourself
- Which of the myths on this page have you heard before?
- Will you recognise a myth when you hear one?
- Will you be able to give a child the correct information instead?

What every teacher needs to know about HIV and AIDS

Ideas for the classroom

What myths do your pupils believe?

Make a list of ten myths about HIV that you have heard. Use your list to make up a test for your class. Each question should be a statement about HIV or AIDS. Ask the children whether the statement is true or false.

Score the test to see what myths the pupils believe.
Make sure you give your class the correct information afterwards.

Helpful hints

When your pupils say things you know to be incorrect, make sure you challenge them and give the correct information instead. If what they say goes unchallenged, other pupils may believe them and act accordingly.

Remember that it is your duty as a teacher to teach accurately about HIV and AIDS.

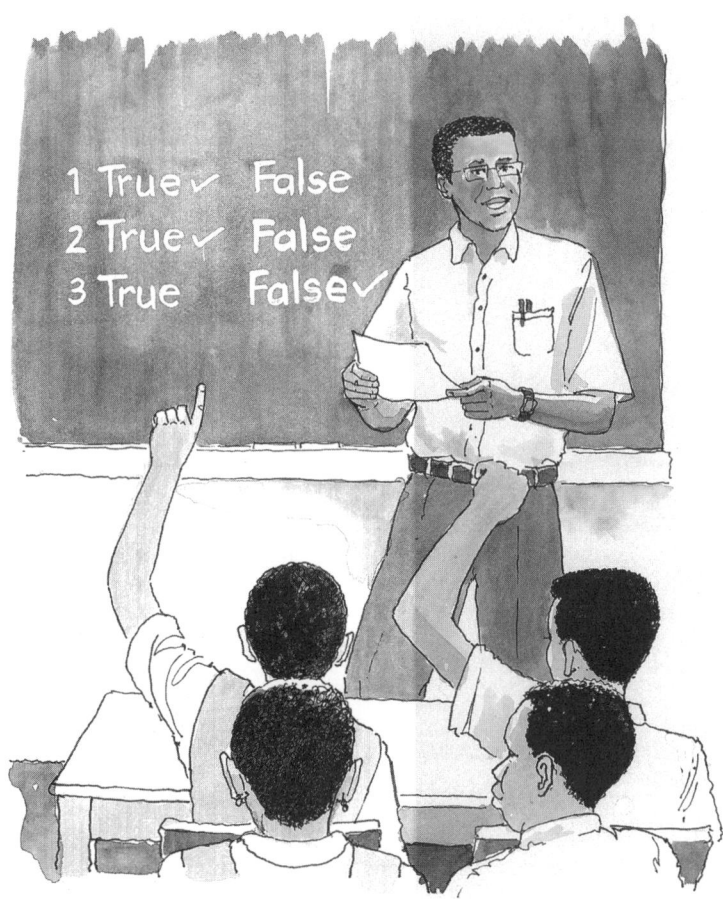

7 Some cultural practices and social conditions encourage HIV to spread

Definitions

Cultural practices are the traditions, customs and habits of people in a society.

Social conditions include poverty, violence and family breakdown that may have an impact on behaviour.

Sexually transmitted diseases (STDs) are infections that spread through sexual contact.

In African societies there are many conditions that allow HIV to spread quickly. Some of these are part of local culture while others are linked to social problems such as poverty, sexual violence or the breakdown of family life. It is important for teachers to understand how the way of life of a community can encourage the spread of HIV.

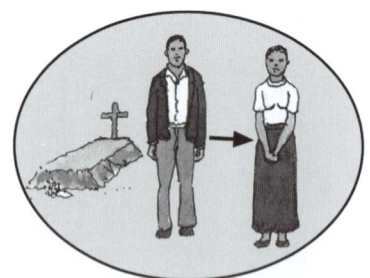

Some cultural practices that encourage the spread of HIV

- **Widow/widower inheritance**
  If a death in the family is caused by AIDS, the widow or widower could be infected with HIV, too. If the widow or widower has unprotected sex with other members of the family, HIV will spread.

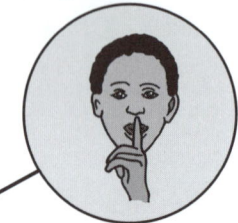

- **Silence and cultural taboos around sexuality**
  These make it hard to teach children accurate information about the link between sex and HIV. As a result, many young people become infected with HIV without realising it.

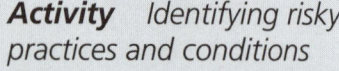

- **Circumcision**
  This can spread HIV if the instruments are not sterilised and if the boys or girls who are circumcised have contact with each other's blood.

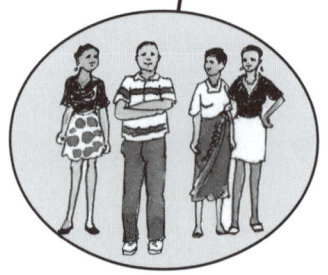

- **Polygamy or multiple sexual partners**
  Having more than one sexual partner increases the risk of spreading HIV.

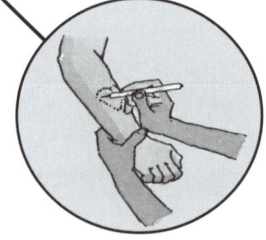

- **Tattooing**
  If sharp instruments are not sterilised completely, blood can enter another person's body and spread HIV.

Activity   Identifying risky practices and conditions

Think about the cultural practices and social conditions in your community that make it easy for HIV to spread. These questions will help you.

- What cultural practices put people at risk of getting HIV? What social conditions influence the practices?
- Are young people under pressure to experiment sexually? How does poverty influence the situation? What social problems help to spread HIV? Do people get HIV because they were raped or molested?

Record your information in the form of 'mind maps' like the ones shown on these pages.

What every teacher needs to know about HIV and AIDS

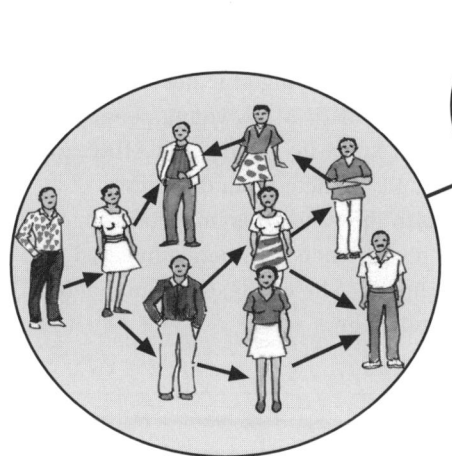

Some social conditions that encourage the spread of HIV
Family breakdown and poverty may lead, for example, to problems such as those shown in these pictures.

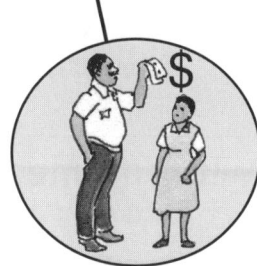

- **Casual sexual relationships outside marriage**
These relationships often involve unprotected sex, and with each sexual contact there is a high risk of becoming infected with HIV.

- **'Sugar daddies' (and 'mummies')**
In many places it has become common for older men to turn to younger girls for sex, because they believe girls are free of HIV. These older men have more power than the girls and this makes it difficult for them to say 'no' or to insist on using condoms. Sometimes, girls like to have older 'sugar daddies', who pay their school fees or buy them clothes in exchange for sex. Older women can also be involved with adolescent boys in this way. Just like men having sex with girls under the age of consent, this is wrong. Moreover, older women, just like older men, may have had many sex partners. This increases the risk of being infected with HIV.

Ideas for the classroom

Many girls are expected to be submissive to men. They also often depend on men for money. This makes them more vulnerable to HIV infection. You can help boys and girls to think about this problem. Divide the class into groups so that the girls can work on their own, and the boys can do the same. Ask every group to do a visual 'mind map' (like the example on page 16) about the things in their communities which make it easier for HIV to spread.

Use the mind map on that and this page and the pupils' own mind maps to start a class discussion about how to make the world a safer place for young people, especially girls. (See also Topic 40, page 86.)

Activity

Read through the 'Ideas for the classroom' again, and think about the ways in which girls become vulnerable to HIV as a result of being expected to be submissive. But can you think of ways in which boys who are encouraged to be aggressive might also make themselves vulnerable?

Helpful hints

- Be critical but fair. Do not apologise for harmful or irresponsible behaviour, even if it is traditional or widespread. (See also Topic 16, page 34.)
- Speak up for community activities that can help to prevent the spread of HIV, such as women's groups.

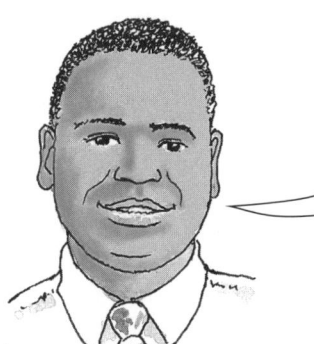

Socio-economic problems, such as poverty and unemployment can contribute to the spread of HIV. When people are desperate, they will have sex so they can get money or food.

Many women and girls are vulnerable because of sexual violence, such as rape and child abuse. All these problems increase if there is a war or a drought. This makes it a very complicated problem for our communities to solve.

8 Living positively with HIV

Definition

People with HIV can get **opportunistic infections** like skin diseases, TB, pneumonia and cancer. Opportunistic infections occur when germs take advantage of the weak immune system to invade the body and make it sick. A healthy diet and good medical care help to prevent opportunistic infections.

Developing a positive attitude

Teaching about HIV and AIDS in Africa has to go further than talking about ways of preventing the spread of HIV. Many young people are already infected, even if they do not know it yet. HIV and AIDS education is an important opportunity to help them develop a positive attitude towards living with the virus. It is important to realise also that during the first phase when a person is infected with HIV but not showing symptoms, he/she can lead a completely normal life, working, studying, and so on.

Living positively with HIV means:

1 Looking after the body

Take personal hygiene seriously to avoid getting ill.

Go to a health worker if you have any unusual symptoms such as unexpected weight loss, diarrhoea or fevers.

Eat nutritious food such as beans, fish, green leaf vegetables and fruit. All these help the immune system.

Stop smoking and drinking alcohol, because these habits make it harder for the immune system to work.

Get early and correct treatment for all illnesses. Test for TB and get it treated if necessary.

Take daily medication to prevent opportunistic infections.

Use antiretroviral drugs, if they are prescribed by a health worker.

Do some exercise to keep fit, but also take time to rest.

2 Looking after one another

If you are sexually active, always use condoms, or express your sexuality in ways that do not involve sexual intercourse.

Take universal precautions to avoid contact with blood. (See Topic 3, pages 8–9.)

Talk to your sexual partner about your HIV infection and find ways to make love safely.

Take time to be with people you love.

Talk about your feelings and about your worries so people know how to support you.

Take part in family functions and community events.

3 Thinking about making the best of life

Talk to a friend or a counsellor to get support with emotional problems.

Take time to nurture your spiritual life.

Talk to others who are living with HIV.

Have a positive attitude towards life, without guilt, self-pity and blame.

Continue working as long as possible.

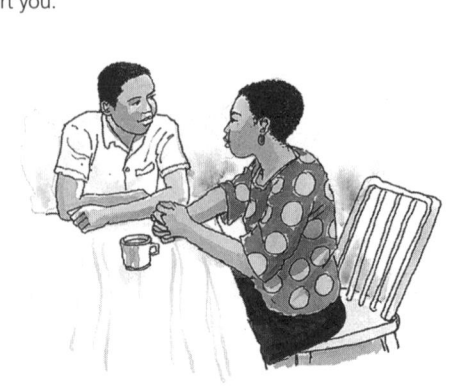

4 Looking after the future

Set a goal or a project you want to achieve.

Make plans for the future.

Help your family to understand your illness and how they can help.

Make sure all your children have their births registered and have applied for social support where possible.

Make a will and talk about funeral arrangements.

What every teacher needs to know about HIV and AIDS

> ### *Activity* Plan a lesson
>
> Look at the box on living positively on the opposite page. Choose one of the headings, 1–4, and plan a lesson on it.
> - How will you introduce the topic?
> - How will you find out what the pupils already know?
> - How will you create a feeling of trust and openness in the class?

Foods that can cause problems

- Sugar: sugar helps bacteria and fungus to grow, especially the fungus that causes candida or thrush.
- Fried food: cooked oils are hard to digest and can cause stomach problems, especially if a person is suffering from diarrhoea.
- Very spicy food: spices can irritate the stomach and cause diarrhoea.

People living with HIV need a healthy and balanced diet. This includes food rich in protein, like meat, chicken or fish. Beans, peas or lentils also give the body protein, especially when they are mixed with uncooked sunflower oil and eaten with rice.

A healthy diet includes fruits such as bananas, apples, oranges, guavas and avocado. It is good to eat vegetables like tomatoes, carrots and pumpkin, and plenty of green vegetables like spinach, cabbage, peas and beans.

Sometimes people with HIV lose their appetite and do not feel like eating at all. In this case it helps to eat smaller amounts more often. Instead of eating three meals a day, they could try six smaller snacks a day.

Did you know?

A runny stomach causes weight loss and dehydration. The best way to treat diarrhoea is to replace the fluid and the nutrients you have lost. Drink rehydration fluid after every time you have been to the toilet. You can mix your own rehydration fluid, using this recipe:

One cup of clean (boiled) water
Two teaspoons of sugar
A quarter teaspoon of salt
The juice of one freshly squeezed orange.

What kinds of medicines does a person with AIDS need?

- Medicines which help a person with AIDS cope, like soothing ointments and painkillers.
- Medicines for treating opportunistic infections. (These help a person with AIDS recover from an opportunistic infection but do not treat the HIV infection.)
- Antiretrovirals: these help the body to fight HIV. They can help a person with AIDS live longer but are not a complete cure.

It is important to take the **right** medicines, in the **right** amounts and at the **right** time. Only take medicines that are prescribed by a trained health worker and follow the instructions faithfully.

Ideas for the classroom

- Teach the children how to live with people who are HIV positive.
- Teach them about nutrition and how to cook meals that boost the immune system. Give them recipes to try.
- Encourage them to practise universal precautions (see Topic 3, pages 8–9, for more information).
- Share ideas about how to show love and compassion in the family.
- Encourage children to ask questions about HIV and how it could affect their life.

Helpful hint

Encourage the children to treat HIV positive people with love, care and understanding. The key message is that people with HIV can remain well for many years. They need our support and care.

9 Caring for people with AIDS

> **Definitions**
>
> **Compassion** is the ability to understand the suffering of other people.
>
> **Empathy** is a life skill that helps us to be compassionate.

In many communities, people with AIDS are young adults who were full of energy and had made exciting plans for their lives. Now their lives have become full of sickness, anger, fear and grief. Families who expected to plan weddings are now attending funerals and many grandparents are caring for their children and grandchildren at a time in their lives when they had hoped to have a rest.

The courage to care

It takes a lot of courage to care for someone who has AIDS. Our communities need people with compassion for others and people who are able to respond to the physical and emotional needs of families affected by AIDS.

If you are a care-giver, you could be doing many different things. In some situations, you will have to shop and cook. In others, you will listen and pray. Sometimes you will clean, or bring medicines, or take a message, or read a book. It always means showing love and kindness. It always means being a friend.

When you give physical care and support to a person with AIDS, it is important to practise universal precautions (see pages 8–9). This involves wearing strong plastic gloves when you touch body fluids that contain HIV. Also wear gloves if you can when you wash their clothes, change soiled bedclothes or clean away vomit or blood.

Other ways of providing care and support are cooking healthy food, helping people to get to the hospital or clinic when they are sick, helping them to take medication and making sure they have safe drinking water.

Remember that many children are carers, and teachers can help them by giving them information and by encouraging them to develop the skills they need.

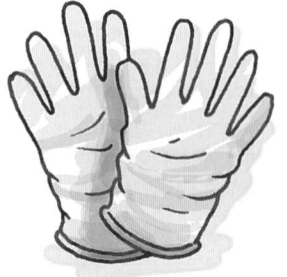

Strong rubber or plastic gloves are very useful when caring for a person infected with HIV.

> **Activity** Reflect on these questions and discuss them with a friend
>
> - Imagine one of your friends or relatives had AIDS. What would be most difficult for you?
> - What do you think would be most difficult for the person with AIDS?

> *When should I wash my hands?*
>
> - Before and after handling food.
> - Before and after feeding or eating.
> - After working with any body fluids or handling bedding and clothes with body fluids on them.
> - Before and after cleaning wounds, bed-sores or any injuries.
> - After removing gloves.
> - After touching animals.
> - After doing any cleaning.
> - After visiting the toilet.
>
> Keeping our hands clean is an important way of reducing infections. This is especially important when we are caring for people with HIV and AIDS. This helps prevent opportunistic infections. (See Topic 8, page 18.)

What every teacher needs to know about HIV and AIDS

I have found that the most important part of caring is to give emotional support. When my sister was at home, sick with AIDS, she knew I could not make her better, but she did not want to be alone. She wanted me to listen to her feelings, but she also asked me to tell her what was on my mind.

At first, I was shy to tell her how angry I was that she got sick. I blamed her for all our problems. But I realised that I had to look at my own fear before I could reach out to her. I remembered what a kind person she is and that anybody can get HIV.

I no longer blame her, but am happy for the time we still have together. Now we talk openly and honestly about our feelings and talking makes us feel less lonely and afraid. Together we have learnt so much about what it means to live with AIDS.

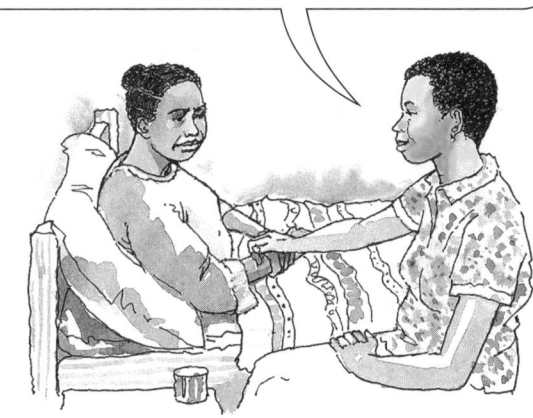

Did you know?

It is very important for people to be touched in a loving way. Hugging, kissing and cuddling can all help to make a person with HIV feel better. Human touch helps our bodies to fight disease.

Ideas for the classroom

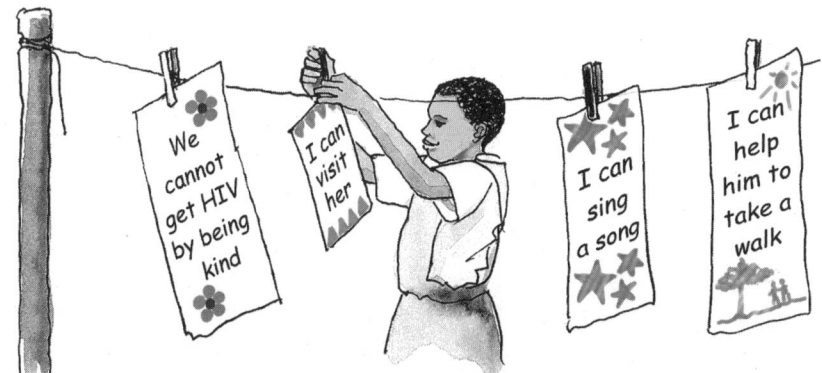

Encourage children to think of practical, everyday ways in which they can show compassion to people living with AIDS.

Put up a 'washing line' in your class and bring some pegs to school. Peg the key message onto the line: *We cannot get HIV by being kind!*

Give the children a piece of paper and ask them to write a beautiful message about how to show love and kindness to a person living with AIDS.

Help them with some ideas, such as 'I can talk to her.' 'I can help him take a walk.' 'I can visit her and tell her what is happening at the market.' 'I can sing him a song.'

When the children have completed their message, let them read it out to the rest of the class and then hang it on the line.

Keep the messages up in class to remind everyone to be kind.

Helpful hints

Before the children write their messages, talk to them about the effects of AIDS. Collect some ideas about what people with AIDS might need.

Encourage children to decorate their message and make it look like a beautiful greeting card.

By expecting good quality work, you are giving them the feeling that their message is important.

10 How HIV and AIDS affect our communities and schools

The wider effects of AIDS

For many communities, AIDS is not only a disease. It is part of their social reality and it changes the way people live and work. It hurts individual people, but it hurts their families too. The families are part of the community. When the families struggle, the community feels the impact of the disease. The case study shows how AIDS changes communities and how this, in turn, affects the schools.

Case study

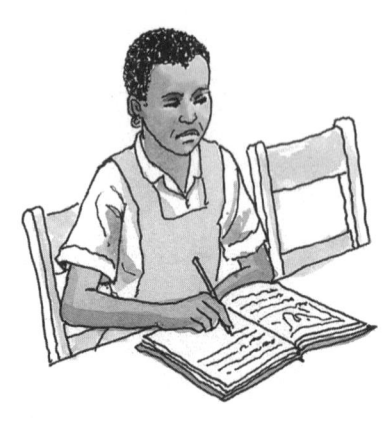

Akuma is twelve years old. She has been attending Domeafa Primary since she started school.

In the last few years, many people in her community have started to suffer from AIDS. This has affected the community badly. Last year, for example, Akuma's teacher died in the middle of the year.

For the last few months she had no teacher and so she did not do well at school. Now she is worried her father will stop her education and send her out to work.

Akuma's friend Grace already is out of school this year. Grace's father died and her mother is now very ill. Grace and her younger sisters have to take care of her. The neighbours and family do not really want to help because they mistakenly believe they could get AIDS if they get involved.

Now Grace has to cook and work in the coffee fields. It is hard work. She tries her best to get money, but the family has little left to sell.

Activity   How did AIDS change life at Domeafa?

Discuss how AIDS changed life at in Domeafa.

How does Akuma's story relate to your own experience?

AIDS and education

When there is AIDS in a community, the quality of education is affected. This can happen in several ways.

- Family members are ill and die. This leaves children orphaned and many drop out of school to make a living. As a result the general level of education in the community drops.
- When many people are ill, they cannot work and they grow less food. This means many families are getting poorer and their children come to school hungry. This makes it difficult to concentrate and learn.
- Many people are in shock, or they are grieving because they have lost someone they love. Many children will feel depressed or disturbed. Children affected by HIV and AIDS are children with special educational needs.
- Teachers become ill and die. This makes it difficult to run an efficient school.

What every teacher needs to know about HIV and AIDS

> **Activity** Think about or discuss how HIV and AIDS have affected your school
> - Have many children dropped out of school?
> - Are the children in school affected by AIDS?
>
> (See also Section 6, pages 108–129.)

Ideas for the classroom

You can help children to understand how HIV and AIDS can affect their lives. Here are some ideas.

Read Akuma and Grace's stories to the class and ask them to compare their experience with their own.

Suggest they use Akuma and Grace's stories to make up short plays about children affected by HIV.

Divide the class into two groups. One group will make up and present a short play showing a day in the life of Akuma and Grace before AIDS made people ill. The other group will present a short play about Akuma and Grace now that so many people are ill. Allow each group to present their scene. Talk about the two scenes. What is similar? What is different? What is the biggest change caused by AIDS?

Finally, ask each pupil to write down a 'message' for the plays they presented.

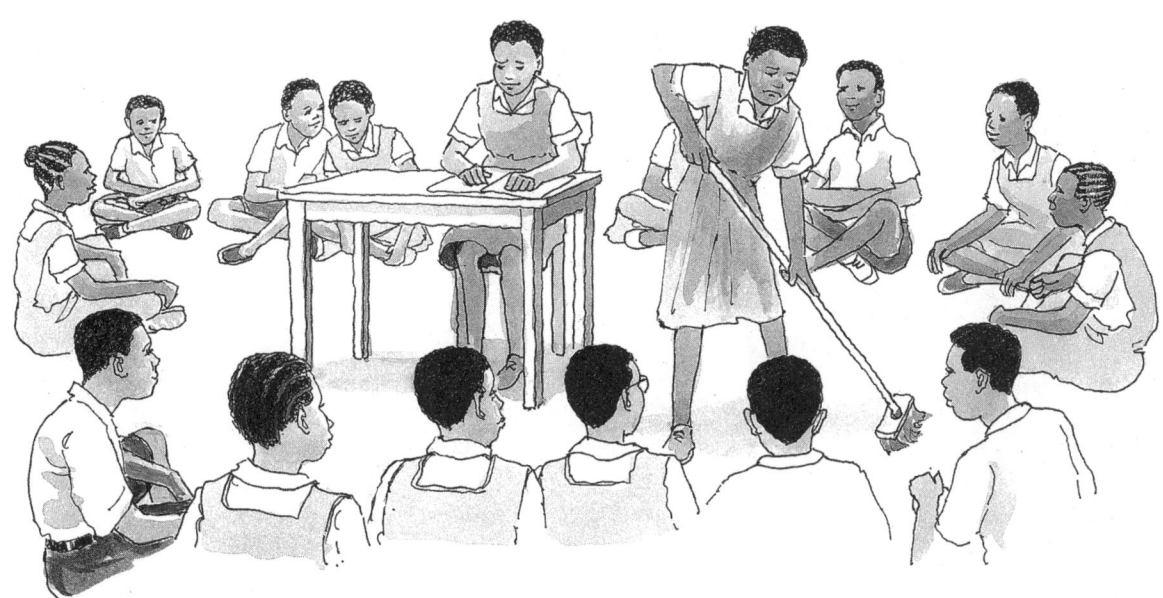

A play about Akuma and Grace

- Give the children a clear time-frame, so they know how long they have to plan their presentation, when they can practise it and how long the final scene must be.
- Encourage the groups to be creative and entertaining. Some children might feel very upset about the way AIDS affects their lives. Respect their feelings. Show compassion by listening to what they have to say.

(See also Topic 18, page 38, *Education can help prevent the spread of HIV and AIDS*.)

11 Sex and the teacher

In most countries, it is against the law for adults to have sex with children under the age of 16 or 18. It is called defilement, sexual abuse or statutory rape.

An adult responsibility

The law against having sex with children exists because children are not yet emotionally mature enough to make decisions about sexual relationships with adults. They are dependent on them, and do not have the power or skills to resist sexual pressure. Sex between children and adults is an abuse of power and will harm a child, even if the child encourages it or is willing. The responsibility for sex between child and adult is always the adult's.

Activity *Who is to blame?*

Although it is against the law, and against the teachers' codes of practice, many teachers still have sex with their pupils. Look at this picture.

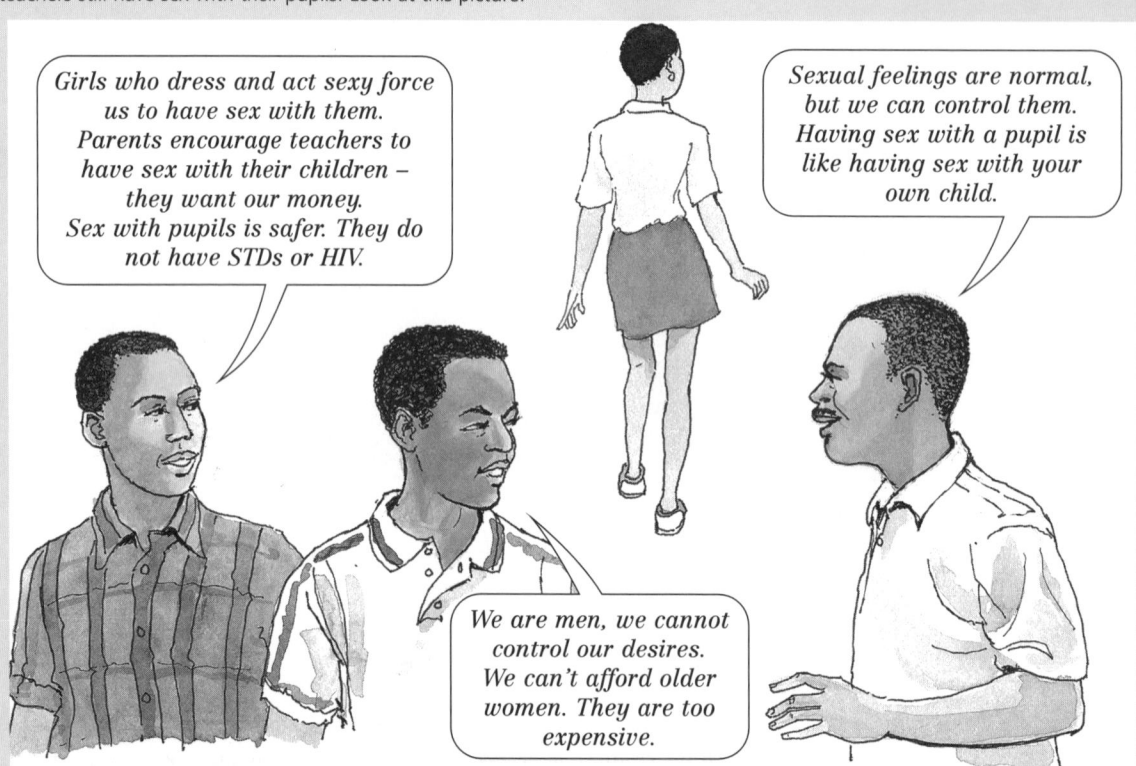

- What do you think about the reasons that one teacher gives for not having sex with pupils? Are they good reasons?
- What do you think about the reasons that these teachers give for having sex with pupils? Who and what are they blaming? Are there any examples of 'Blaming the victim'? Are they taking responsibility for their own actions?
- Find out who or what else teachers blame for having sex with their pupils. An unhappy marriage? A low salary? Girls who are already sexually mature?

This material is based on an extract from Teacher Talk, *published by the Straight Talk Foundation, Uganda*

What every teacher needs to know about HIV and AIDS

> ### Blaming the victim
>
> Blaming the person who is being abused is called 'Blaming the Victim'.
>
> An example is when girls who are used to satisfy the sexual feelings of adults are punished again by society. They are called names like 'prostitutes' or 'loose women' and often are forced to stop schooling if, for example, they get pregnant. This can make them dependent and open to being abused again.

Taking responsibility

Here are some messages to help teachers take responsibility for their actions and to stop them from having sex with pupils. They are taken from *Teacher Talk*, an HIV and AIDS magazine for teachers.

- There are never any excuses to have sex with children, even if pupils are already sexually active themselves.
- Sexual feelings are normal but they do not have to lead to sex. It is your responsibility to control them!
- Some pupils will want to have sex with you. Always say 'No'!
- Even if the pupils are willing to have sex with you it is wrong!
- Never give in to parents who want to convince you to have sex with their children! Sex with a child is a crime.
- Pupils are not always free from HIV! Some children can be born with HIV, and others may have had sexual experiences.
- Be brave. Problems are no excuse for having sex with a pupil. If you are lonely, unhappy or have financial difficulties, get help from friends or religion.
- You, as a teacher, are a parent to the pupil and you are responsible for the child. If you have sex with a child, you are betraying him or her.

Ideas for the classroom

Talk to children about having sexual feelings for teachers. Remind them about the difference between infatuation and love (see Topic 26, page 56). Explain that they can only have a healthy sexual relationship with a teacher once they are much older, adult and out of school.

Do a role-play to practise saying 'No!' to a teacher's advances. Anna Assertive (see Topic 28, page 61 and Topic 30, page 65) can be the pupil and you could act the role of a handsome new teacher who promises to give her good marks in exchange for a kiss. Make the story appropriate for the age of the children.

> ### Helpful hints
>
> Girls and boys are often attracted to their teachers and may want to have a sexual relationship with you. This is a normal and healthy part of their sexual development.
>
> Part of your job is **never** to give in or to respond to sexual pressure from your pupils. Some may even threaten you or say that they will hurt themselves if you do not agree to have sex with them. When this happens, you can do the following.
>
> - Treat the pupil with respect and never humiliate them.
> - Tell them that it is against the law and against your principles for a teacher to have a relationship with a pupil.
>
> If you find out that one of your colleagues is having a sexual relationship with a pupil, it is important that you speak to the principal immediately. If the principal does not follow it up, find out from the education department officials where you could report this. It is generally better if a group of teachers report the matter together. This can stop one teacher from being victimised.

Section 2 Laying the foundations – understanding our attitudes to HIV and AIDS

12 What it means to live with HIV and AIDS

Definitions

Emotional support means helping someone feel cared for and loved. This can be done by being there, listening and comforting a person in need.

Disclosure means telling people that you have HIV or AIDS.

Teachers with HIV and AIDS

Have any of the teachers at your school disclosed that they have HIV or AIDS? How did the school respond? If this has not happened yet, how do you think your school would respond if a teacher told that they have HIV or AIDS? Here is a story of a teacher who had to cope with having AIDS.

Case study

Mrs Taylor has been teaching in her village school for 35 years. She is loved and respected in the community. In the last year she has often been sick. She gets very tired at school and cries easily.

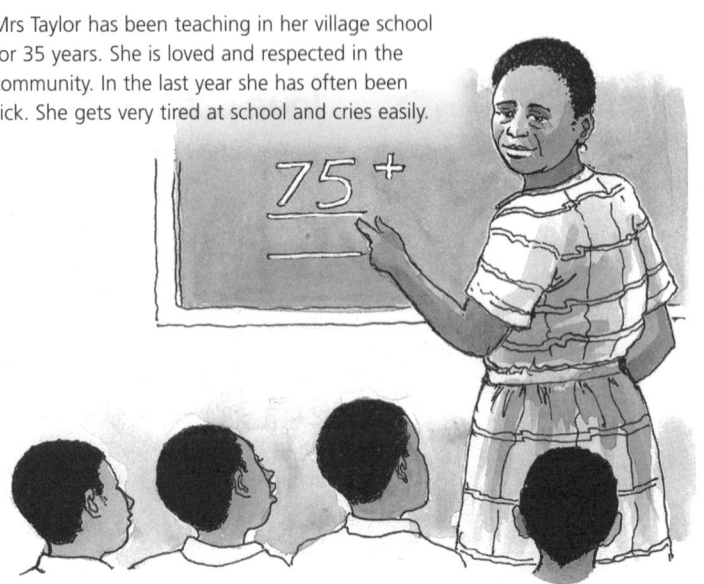

Nobody knows that Mrs Taylor has AIDS. Her husband died two years ago from the sickness. They never had any children. Mr Taylor had always been a gentle man but, before he died, he changed. He was angry and drank a lot. When he came home he cried and wanted to have sex with her. One night he told her that he was infected with HIV. She never asked him about how he had got infected. She thinks that he had sex with another woman when he worked in the city for two years.

Mrs Taylor feels that she can't tell anybody about her illness. There is one woman in the village who told everybody that she has AIDS. Nobody in the village speaks to her. They say that a woman who has HIV or AIDS is a prostitute. Some children shout at her. Mrs Taylor would like to visit her but she is too afraid that someone will see her.

Some of the younger teachers feel that Mrs Taylor should resign. They say that she is getting old and lazy and they are tired of looking after her classes.

Activity Looking at the case study

- How has reading this story made you feel?
- How do you think you would feel, if you found out that you have HIV?
- Why do you think Mrs Taylor did not ask her husband how he got infected?
- If you were in Mrs Taylor's shoes, could you tell your school that you have AIDS? How would you like your school to respond?

Laying the foundations – understanding our attitudes to HIV and AIDS

Activity HIV quiz

Do you think that the people in your community have correct information about teachers living with HIV? Do this quiz to find out. Answer each question as 'T' (true) or 'F' (false).

1 A teacher with HIV must not do exercise or carry anything heavy.
2 It is not healthy for a teacher with HIV to continue to teach.
3 A teacher with HIV has to be careful not to sneeze or cough.
4 A teacher with HIV needs to use a special toilet.
5 A teacher with HIV should stay away from children who are sick.
6 A teacher with HIV must not hug children in her class too much.

(The answers are on page 130.)

AIDS in the school

For a school, living with AIDS can mean coping with colleagues and pupils who are often ill, tired and depressed. Teachers may have to take on extra classes and do more work. This can cause anger and frustration. The story of Mrs Taylor shows how important it is to have knowledge and understanding of AIDS. Without this it is very difficult to help sick people.

How a teacher with HIV should live

A teacher with HIV can lead a happy and productive life. This means eating healthy food, doing exercise, resting and looking after yourself and feeling that you are contributing something to society for as long as possible. When an infected teacher is ill, she or he should be treated like any other sick teacher.

A teacher with HIV has to be careful not to catch sickness from others because his or her resistance to infection is lower. The whole school must practise good hygiene. For example, people should hold a hand in front of the nose and mouth when coughing or sneezing.

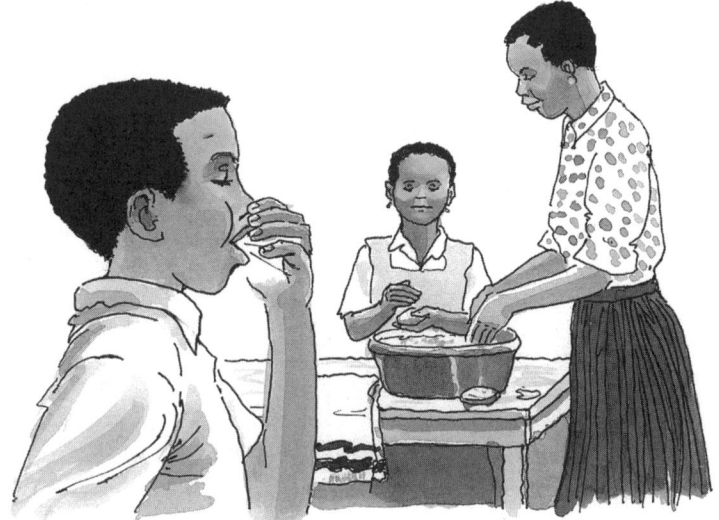

People should not spit, because this can spread illness, such as tuberculosis. Everybody should be encouraged to wash their hands regularly. (See also Topic 9, page 20.)

Ideas for the classroom

Children need to learn that illness is part of life. They also need to see that sick people, especially those suffering from AIDS, should be treated with kindness.

Let pupils talk, write or draw a picture about when they were ill. Discuss what others did to make them feel better and what others did that made them feel worse. They can talk about what it would be like to be ill often and to know that you may never get better. Discuss what a friend who has AIDS might need from us.

Helpful hint

As a teacher, it is important to keep yours ears open for stories you can tell your pupils. Stories are a powerful way to look at difficult topics. There are many that help children deal with death and illness.

13 Helping teachers look at their own risk

> *Definition*
>
> **Confidential** means no one will be told.

As adults who teach about HIV and AIDS, it is important to think about and know whether we have been infected with HIV ourselves. The only way to know is to go for a test.

Reasons to take an HIV test

There are several reasons why you may not want to go for an HIV test. For example, you may not feel ready, or you may never have had sex.

However, there are good reasons to take an HIV test. Firstly, if you know that you do not have HIV, it can make you feel better and motivate you to stay safe in future. Secondly, if you know you do have HIV, you can make sure that you do not infect others. You can also find out how to stay healthy for longer. It sets a good example to others and shows courage to face up to the disease.

> *Am I at risk?*
>
> If any of these statements are true for you, you may have HIV, and it is better to have a test.
>
> - I can't remember who I had sex with in the last five years.
> - I have had unprotected sex with more than one person in the last three years.
> - My partner says that she or he would never take an HIV test.
> - My partner likes to make me feel bad and does not listen to me.
> - My partner believes it is his or her right to have sex with me.
> - My partner says she or he will never have sex with a condom.
> - My partner has had other partners.
> - Sometimes I get drunk and have unprotected sex.
> - I have been to a traditional healer who cut me with a knife or blade used on others.
> - I have helped people who are bleeding without wearing protection.
>
> If you decide not to go for a test, there are things you can do to protect others and yourself. (See Topics 24–27, pages 50–59.)

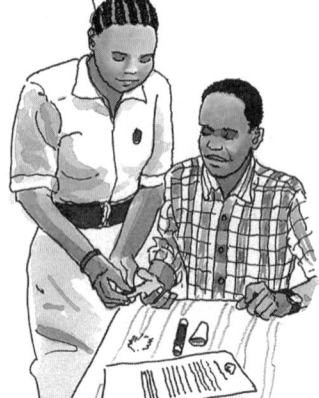

Getting tested

It is useful to know about HIV testing so that you can answer any questions in the classroom about it. Children need to know that testing is an important part of preventing the spread of HIV and AIDS.

Testing is usually done at clinics, hospitals or by private doctors. Blood is taken and tested. The results are normally accurate. If the result shows that you do not have HIV, it is important to go for testing again in three months time to make sure you are not in the **window period** (see Topic 2, page 4). The results are confidential. No one is allowed to tell anyone about the results without your permission.

Laying the foundations – understanding our attitudes to HIV and AIDS

Activity *Should I disclose that I have HIV?*

Read these comments about whether or not someone should disclose that they have HIV. Discuss them with your colleagues.

- 'I think you should tell as many people as possible that you have HIV. It helps them to see that the disease is real. It can teach them to be more careful.'
- 'Disclosure will hurt your family and friends. Everybody will point a finger at you and your family.'
- 'I think you must be careful who you tell. I wouldn't want my small children to know what their mother died of. They will suffer.'
- 'I prefer to be honest with my children and my family. It means they won't find out through gossip what is happening to me. It also gives them a chance to help me when I need them.'

Counselling

It is best to get counselling before and after you are tested. Counsellors can help, whether the results are positive or negative.

A counsellor may ask you to think about these questions.

- Who can I talk to if I find out that I have HIV?
- What is the first thing I will do if I find out that I have HIV?
- If I find out that I do not have HIV, how will I reduce my risk of getting it?

(For advice, see Topics 24–27, pages 50–59.)

Ideas for the classroom

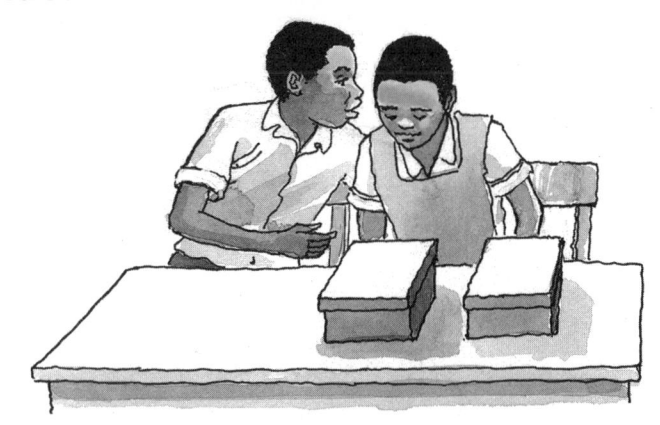

To introduce the topic of disclosure to pupils, you could speak to them about keeping secrets. Show them two closed boxes. Tell them that each one contains a secret. The secrets are written below. The teacher can take the secrets out of the boxes, or the pupils can volunteer to do so.

Secret 1
John's mother has told him that he is going to get a beautiful new pair of shoes. She doesn't want him to tell anybody, but he is so happy that he wants to tell you.

Secret 2
Mary's uncle has been touching her private parts. He has said that if she tells anybody he is going to kill her. She is scared of him.

Discuss with the pupils:

- When does keeping a secret harm you and when is it fun?
- How should I respond to a harmful secret? How should I respond to a fun secret?
- Who should I tell my secret to?
- Who could I talk to if I thought that I, or someone I love, might have a sickness like AIDS?

From the discussion, lead the children to talk about testing for HIV. Talk about why and where one could go for testing. It is also useful to let them discuss who they would feel safe talking to if they, or someone they loved, tested positive.

14 Understanding our feelings about HIV and AIDS

Definitions

Denial means not wanting to see that bad things, like AIDS, exist.

Grief means to feel sadness, pain and unhappiness.

How do you think you would react if you found out that someone close to you has HIV or AIDS? Everybody reacts to shock in their own way. Some get angry, some get sad, others start to look for someone to blame.

Reactions and actions

The story of Mrs Taylor and the other woman in her village who had AIDS (see Topic 12, page 26) shows us how our feelings can make us act cruelly towards people who need our support. HIV and AIDS bring with it many strong feelings. It forces us to look at sex, death, illness and the fear of losing those we love. To be able to teach about HIV and AIDS, a teacher needs to have a good knowledge and understanding of feelings.

Activity Look at the picture

The family has just found out that the father has got HIV. Match these feelings to the people in the picture: anger; grief; blaming; sadness; refusing to feel pain. The people can have more than one feeling each.

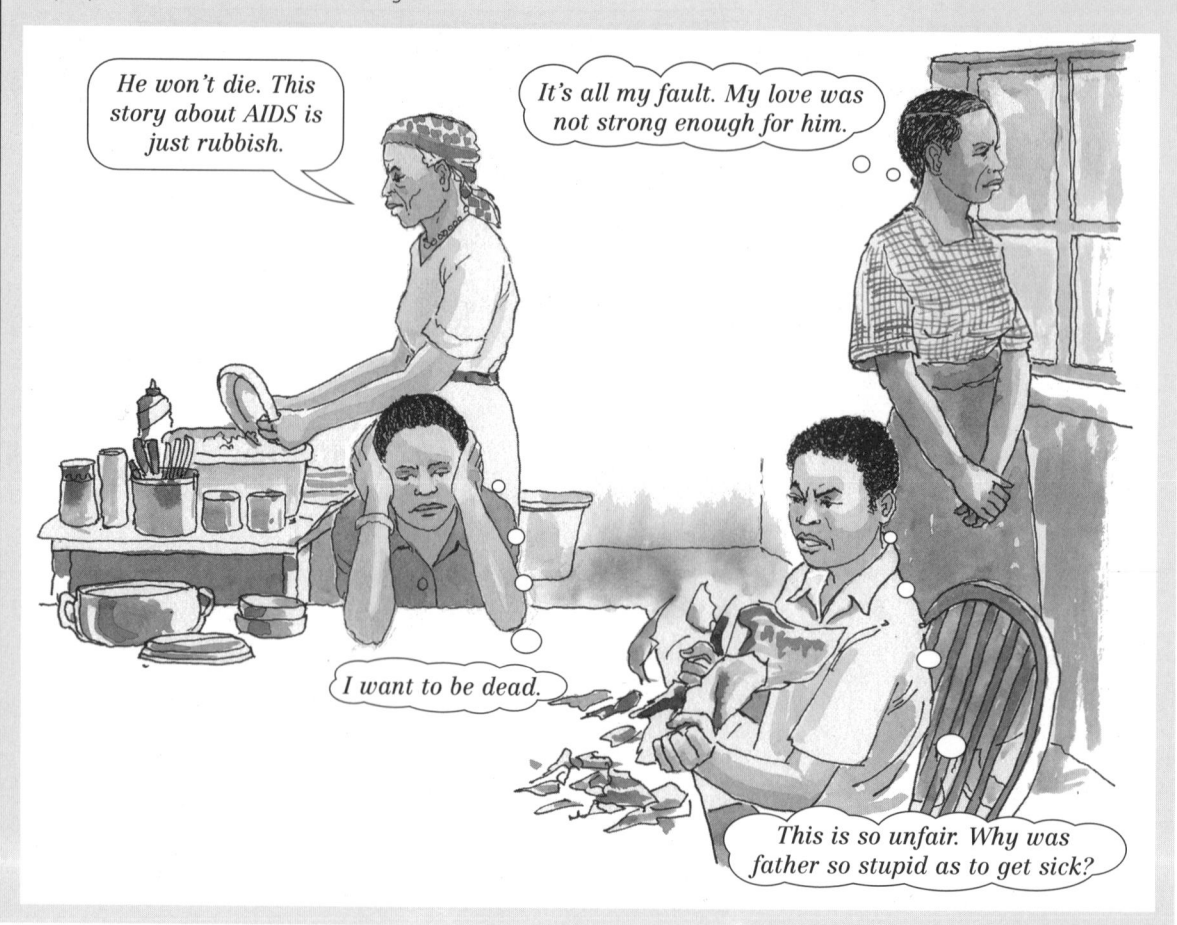

He won't die. This story about AIDS is just rubbish.

It's all my fault. My love was not strong enough for him.

I want to be dead.

This is so unfair. Why was father so stupid as to get sick?

Laying the foundations – understanding our attitudes to HIV and AIDS

Common feelings about AIDS

This family shows some of the most common feelings people have about AIDS. Match these points to the picture of the family opposite.

Look at how the people in the pictures respond to AIDS. Who blames? Who is sad? Who gets angry?

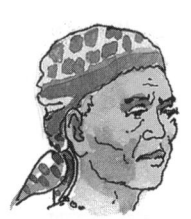

- The grandmother refuses to feel pain and accept that there is a problem. This is something that many people do when they think about AIDS. It is called *denial*. Often, people are in denial because they do not want to face the pain of what is happening.

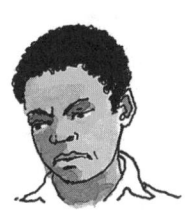

- The son shows his sadness by being angry. He is also looking for someone to blame, someone to be angry with, so that he does not have to feel so much pain.

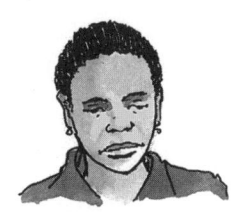

- The daughter is feeling deep grief and sadness. If she stays sad for a long time, it is called a depression.

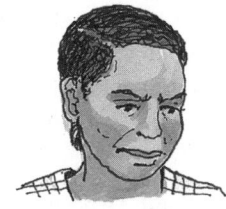

- The mother shows her sadness by blaming herself.

Activity Your responses 1

How do you think you would respond if you found out that you had HIV? Make a list of what you would be most afraid of.

Here are some common fears and thoughts that people have.

- Who did I get HIV from?
- When will I become ill with AIDS?
- Will I suffer?
- Will there be treatment for me?
- What will happen to my family when I die?
- For how long will I live?
- How will people react when I tell them I have HIV?
- Will I be lonely?

Activity Your responses 2

How do you think you would respond if someone in your family had HIV? Make a list of what you would be most afraid of.

Here are some common fears that people have.

- Will I be strong enough to help them?
- Do we have enough money to cope?
- I won't be able to take away their suffering.
- How long will they be ill?
- When will they die?
- How will people react if they find out?
- I will be left alone.

Ideas for the classroom

Help your pupils to learn to understand and talk about feelings. It will help them to understand themselves and others.

Help pupils to collect as many words as they can to describe feelings. Let them give each feeling a colour and a taste and draw pictures about the feelings. You could put these pictures on the walls. Refer to the pictures and words when you are telling stories or when a child is very emotional and does not know how to express it.

They can also collect pictures that show strong emotions, such as a person crying, being very sad or angry. Speak to learners about the feelings shown in the pictures. Let the children discuss in pairs which of these feelings they would have if they found out that someone they love is very sick. Let the partner respond by saying how they would help them to cope with these feelings.

15 Understanding my own attitudes to HIV and AIDS

Definitions

Prejudice means judging someone without really understanding them.

Compassion means feeling and showing that you care and would like to help.

Sympathy means feeling sorry for another person.

To be able to deal with HIV and AIDS at our school and in our community it is important to look at our own attitudes towards people who are living with HIV and AIDS.

Activity How much sympathy do you feel?

Look at the pictures on this page. They show people who are living with HIV. Give each one a score of 1 – 5 for how much sympathy you feel for them. A score of 1 means you have no sympathy, a score of 2 means you have very little sympathy – and so on, up to 5, which means you have a lot of sympathy.

These people are all HIV positive

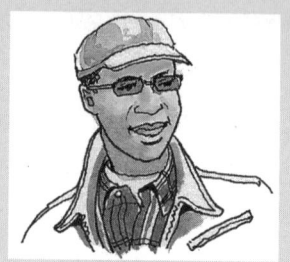

David is a taxi driver.

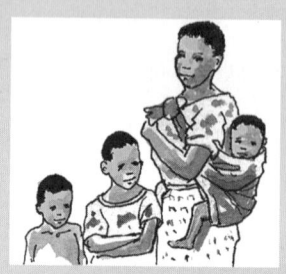

Hanna is a housewife.

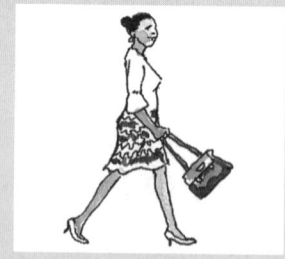

Beryl is a musician.

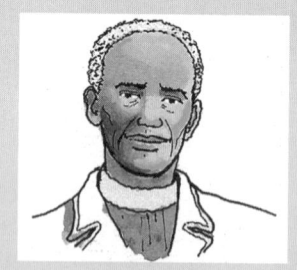

John is a priest.

Write down your sympathy scores on a piece of paper, and then turn to page 130 and find out how each one of these became HIV positive.

Have your sympathies changed?

Did your sympathies for the people in the pictures change when you found out more about them? Why do you think this is so? What does this tell you about your own values and prejudices?

This exercise shows how easy it is to judge people, and we should not do this. We often decide whether others are good or bad before we even know them. Just notice how often in one day you think cruel things about yourself or others. 'I am ugly', 'You are stupid', 'I am too slow' or 'You are not as good as she is'.

The exercise also shows that anyone can get HIV and AIDS. It does not matter how a person got infected. What matters is that we support them.

Remember

We should not fight the people living with HIV and AIDS, but we need to fight the disease instead.

Laying the foundations – understanding our attitudes to HIV and AIDS

Activity

Think about how whether a person's gender makes a difference to your own perception of people with HIV or AIDS. Are you more or less critical or judgmental of women than you are of men – or the other way around?

Ideas for the classroom

Help pupils understand how prejudice can hurt. You could adapt the exercise above to suit your class. Let children discuss how we cannot judge people from the way they look or by their jobs.

For homework, pupils can ask older people in the community for sayings about not judging others and about having compassion. For example: 'You can't judge a book by its cover.' 'Judge not, lest ye be judged.' Make posters of these sayings or quotations and put them up in the classroom.

Ask pupils to think of the last time someone judged them unfairly. Let them tell the story to a partner and then write about or draw what happened. It is important to focus on how it made them feel.

Suggest that pupils write or draw about how they would like to be treated if they had AIDS. Children are naturally compassionate. It is important to encourage this and to make them aware of how hurtful judging can be. To follow on to the lesson about judging others, the children discuss in groups why we should show compassion to people living with AIDS.

The children in the picture below are suggesting reasons why we should be compassionate.

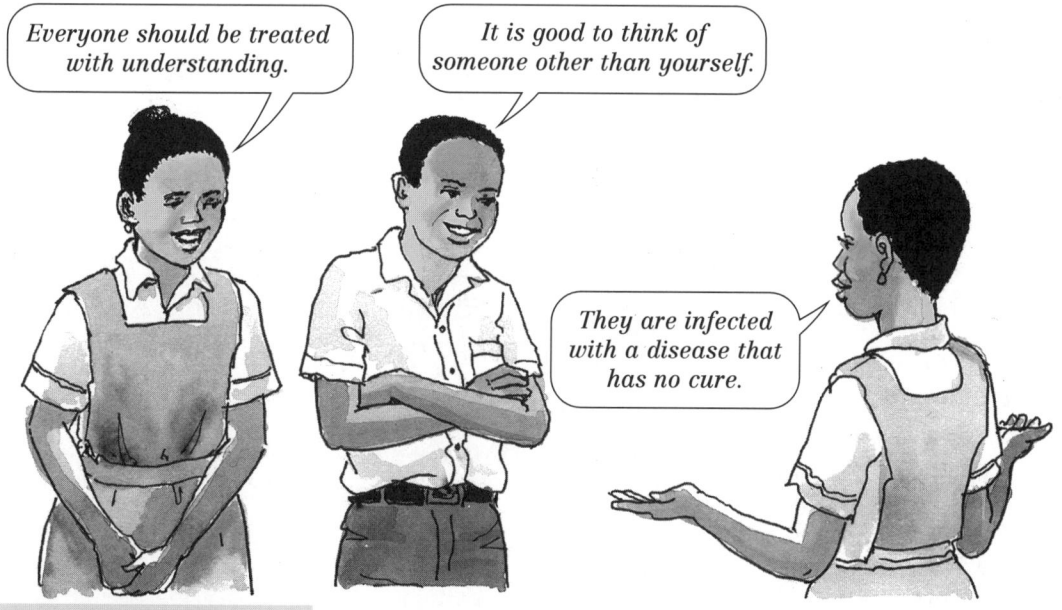

Everyone should be treated with understanding.

It is good to think of someone other than yourself.

They are infected with a disease that has no cure.

Helpful hint

It is important to keep moral judgements separate from our teaching about the facts of HIV and AIDS. Children need to understand that it does not matter much why and how someone got infected with HIV. What does matter is that we care for them.

Ask pupils to think of more reasons why we should be compassionate. Then let them choose the two reasons that they find the most important.

They can also discuss why it is easy for some people to show compassion, and more difficult for others.

16 My community's attitudes towards AIDS

Definition
Helplessness is feeling as if you are not able to do anything about a situation.

Investigating attitudes

Look at the pictures below. Do you recognise any of these responses to AIDS in your community?

AIDS doesn't exist, they just want to scare us.

I don't care about AIDS, as long as I can have fun.

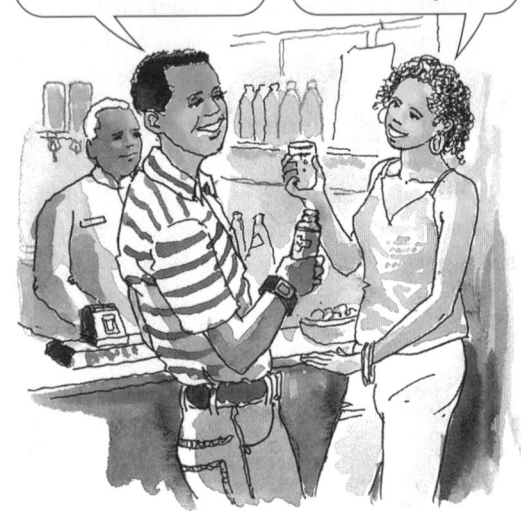

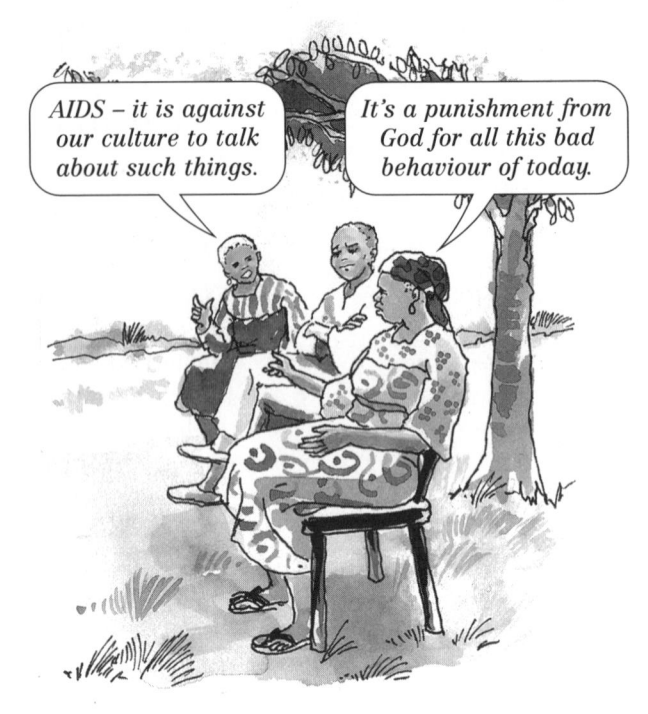

AIDS – it is against our culture to talk about such things.

It's a punishment from God for all this bad behaviour of today.

Helpful and harmful attitudes of a community towards AIDS

Harmful attitudes	Helpful attitudes
Denial: the community ignores its problems.	Openness about the problems in the community.
Fear of any change: even change that can bring good to the community.	Being willing to change if it is for the good of the community.
The community blames everybody else for AIDS.	The community is prepared to look at its own mistakes.
The community does not look after people who are ill with AIDS or the orphans left behind.	The community looks after the ill and after orphans.
The community feels helpless about AIDS and does nothing about it.	The community looks for solutions to its problems.

Activity   Which attitudes are helpful?

Before you can teach about AIDS it is important to understand the attitudes of your own community and to see which attitudes are helpful and which are not. Look at the table with your colleagues and discuss the attitudes.

To help children understand the ideas of community better, it is useful to let them act out the responses of different people. Have a debate between a conservative old man or woman, a young teenager, a wealthy businessman, a poor farmer and a wise man or woman.

Laying the foundations – understanding our attitudes to HIV and AIDS

These characters could respond to situations such as:
1 A leader has died of AIDS and he has no relatives left. The community has to decide whether they should reveal what he has died of.
2 A school has decided to exclude a child because her mother is ill with AIDS.

Activity   More thoughts about attitudes

Look at the table on page 34. Add any more harmful or helpful attitudes you have found in your community to the table.

- What good things can you say about the way your community deals with problems?
- What good things can you say about the way your community deals with AIDS?
- What cultural practices promote the spread of HIV and AIDS in your community? (See Topic 7, pages 16–17, for more ideas.)
- How does your community respond to the things it is afraid of? Does it refuse to speak about these things? Does it look for blame? Is it helpless?
- What social problems is your community silent about? Sexual abuse? Alcohol and drug abuse? Violence against women? Prostitution? Child labour? AIDS?
- Who or what is blamed for AIDS?
- What is your community most afraid of when it comes to dealing with AIDS? Talking openly about sex? Looking at its faults?
- What opportunities do you, as a teacher, have to change dangerous attitudes that can cause AIDS to spread in your community?
- What opportunities does your school have to lead the community in fighting AIDS?

Ideas for the classroom

It is important to make children aware that we get many of our attitudes and ideas from our community. It is also helpful to see whether our own attitudes are useful or not. This is a good introduction to peer pressure, which is discussed later (Topic 30, pages 64–65).

Older children could prepare a debate about whether we always have to obey our elders, or those who lead us, even if we disagree with what they do and say.

Younger children could start discussing when it is right to disagree with an adult. This links with assertiveness and learning to say 'No' (see Topic 28, pages 60–61).

If you have a local newspaper, you could let children cut out pictures and make two collages. They can call one 'What I like about my community' and the other 'What I don't like about my community'. Children could also draw pictures about these two topics.

Helpful hint

It is important to involve the parents and other members of the community in your teaching about HIV and AIDS. This is so that the information can be reinforced outside the school, and so that children can see that AIDS is something that affects everybody. (See also Topic 17, page 37 for more ideas about involving parents in AIDS education.)

17 Our attitudes towards the children we teach

Listening to children

When teaching about emotionally difficult issues such as HIV and AIDS, it is important to look at our attitudes towards children. Do we listen to them? Do we find out how they feel and respect their needs? Do we expect them to keep quiet and obey? Do we make them fear us, so that we can control them or do we build trust?

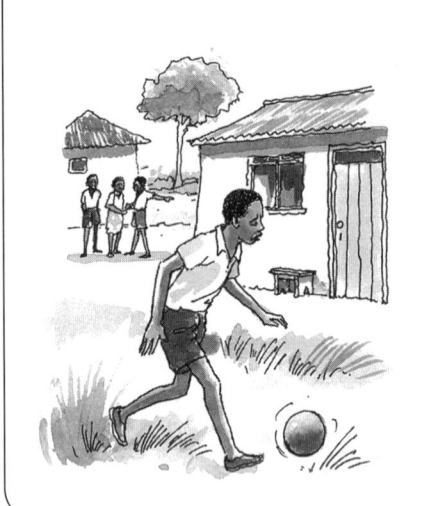

Case study

Thabo lives with his uncle in the village.

Nobody has told him that his mother has died of AIDS. He feels lucky because his uncle can afford to let him go to school. But Thabo misses his mother very much. She was never as strict as his uncle. He used to live with her in town, but two years ago she became very ill and brought him here. Since then, he has not seen her. One day, the neighbour's children began telling him that she was dead.

Thabo gets very angry when anybody says that. When he asks his uncle about it, his uncle pats him on the head and says that she will come back soon. One boy at school said that she was a prostitute and died from AIDS. Thabo hit him hard in the face and his nose started to bleed. His uncle beat him afterwards, but Thabo does not feel bad about what he did.

Every night he prays that God will bring back his mother.

Telling children the truth

How does the story of Thabo in the case study make you feel? Do you think Thabo should have been told about his mother's death?

In many communities, adults find it difficult to speak to children about issues such as death or sex. Some parents live away from their families and do not have the time.

In the past, there were indirect ways in which sex or death were spoken about – for example, through stories; and older adults, such as aunts and grandmothers, talked about these matters during initiation. But societies have changed and, today, some of these ways are lost. There are other reasons too. Thabo's uncle, for example, keeps quiet because he is afraid that Thabo will lose respect and become cheeky. He rules with fear.

Silence can hurt

Thabo's story shows how this silence can hurt children. It can make them lonely and angry. When Thabo finds out that people lied to him about his mother's death, he will find it difficult to trust people in future. He is made powerless by the silence.

Activity *Thinking about attitudes to children*

Do these sayings describe your community's relationship to children?

'We must treat our children well, they are the leaders of the future.'

'Children should be seen and not heard.'

Laying the foundations – understanding our attitudes to HIV and AIDS

This silence can be very dangerous. An angry child will often be rebellious and will not take advice from adults. He or she may do things that are harmful, like having unprotected sex or trying out drugs and alcohol. A child who feels that he or she has no power can become passive and will be easily influenced by others.

Activity   Discussions with parents

Use the story of Thabo to start a discussion with parents about the dangers of silence. They could also think about filling in the gaps in this table.

When I was young:	My child:
I needed more	Needs more ....
I got help from	He/ she can get help from ....
I needed to have been told more about	Needs to be told more about ....

Activity   Thinking back

To understand children, it is important to remember our own childhoods. Here is an activity that you can do on your own in writing, or with colleagues and friends.

- Remember an incident from your childhood when an adult did not listen to you and treated you unfairly. Try to remember the story in as much detail as possible. Where did it happen? What happened? How did it make you feel? How do you think it has influenced your relationships in later life? How has this influenced your teaching?
- Now remember an incident from your childhood when an adult did listen to you and trusted you. Try to remember the story in as much detail as possible. Where did it happen? What happened? How did it make you feel? How do you think it has influenced your relationship to children? How has this influenced your teaching?

Ideas for the classroom

At the beginning of the year, get to know the children in your class by asking them to complete the sentences below. Doing this will also help the pupils to feel better about themselves, and can therefore help to keep them safe. Encourage the children to answer honestly.

My favourite food is ....
My favourite colour is .... because ....
When I am big I want to be ....
I am most afraid of ....
I am happiest when ....
If I could change one thing in the world it would be ....

Think about how you can use the answers to help the children in your class grow strong.

Helpful hints

- When working with children, earn their trust by being honest and caring. Listen carefully to what they say.
- Be patient: it takes time to build good relationships. Allow children to ask questions.
- Remind yourself how a wise and caring adult that you knew as a child would have reacted in your situation.

Section 3 Preventing the spread of HIV and AIDS

18 Education can help prevent the spread of HIV and AIDS

Definition
A **role model** is someone who teaches by the way they act.

Parents are the ones who should teach their children how to stay safe. It isn't the teacher's job.

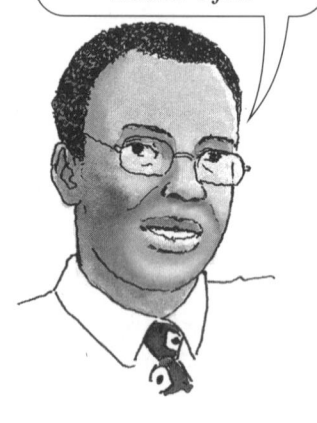

Teaching about AIDS is the job of clinics and nurses.

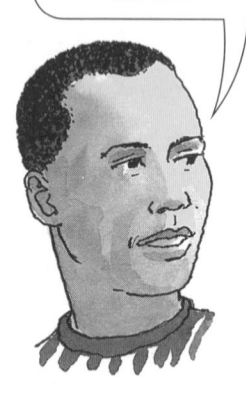

Everybody has to help keep us safe.

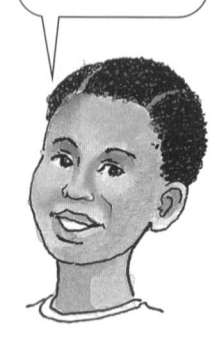

Teachers spend so much time with children, they are the only ones who can help them stay safe.

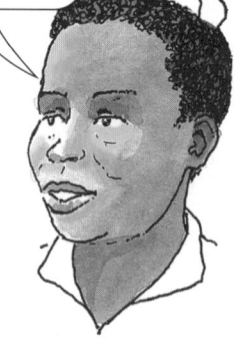

How can education help?

Preventing children from being infected is the most important role of HIV and AIDS education.

The importance of staying at school

Keeping young people at school makes them much less at risk of getting infected with HIV. Education can give knowledge and information about sex and about HIV and AIDS. But, most importantly, it can give young people the skills and motivation to protect themselves.

Being able to read and write can also help people stay safe. It can help them not to get cheated and tricked and to make up their own minds about safe behaviour. It can also make it easier to read instructions, posters and find their way around in a clinic.

Teachers play a very important role in helping young people to stay safe. They can encourage and motivate them. They can act as role models and through their actions show how to be assertive and make positive choices.

Did you know?
Giving young girls an education can help them to protect themselves from HIV. The longer girls stay in school, the longer they can delay sex. Unskilled girls often marry early. Some might have sex in exchange for money. Schooling gives girls more power over their own lives and builds self-esteem. It allows them to have more choices and to use their talents.

Preventing the spread of HIV and AIDS

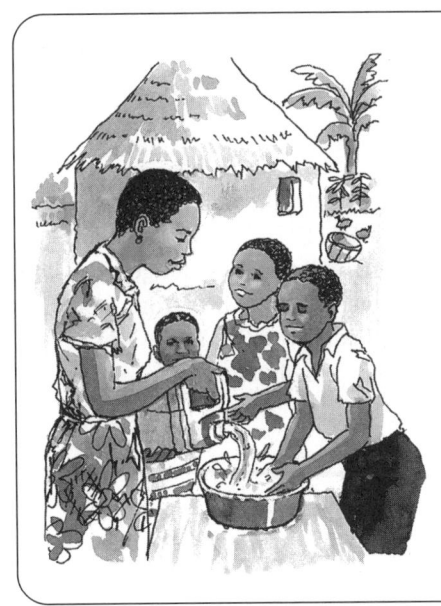

Case study

Why is education so important in helping to prevent the spread of HIV? Here is Martha's story.

Martha used to be the best pupil in her class. She loved to read and to write her own stories. She also enjoyed helping the other children with their homework.

Three years ago, Martha's mother died and left her and her father to look after her younger brothers and sisters. Martha was only thirteen years old then. At first she tried to stay in school but there was too much work. Now she tends the fields and looks after the house. She is often tired and lonely. She misses the time when she used to play with her school friends.

Lately, there have been some men visiting the house. They want to marry a pretty girl like Martha who can work hard. They say nice things to her and she has had sex with one of them. His name is David. Martha does not really like him that much. He drinks and visits many different women. Her father wants her to marry David. He is a lot older than Martha and owns a shop. He brings sugar and other presents from the shop for the family. Nobody knows that David has infected Martha with HIV.

Activity 1   Discuss Martha's story

What do you think will happen next? Do you think that Martha would have been infected with HIV if she had stayed on at school? Could this story have happened at your school? How could the school have made it easier for Martha to stay on? Do you think she would have been infected with HIV if she was a boy?

Activity 2   Discuss Martha's situation

Think about, and discuss, how your school can make it easier for children like Martha not to drop out. Maybe she could be given a place and time during the school day to do her homework. Her classmates could volunteer to help her with her work, especially when she has to miss school.

Think about your own class. Do you know who struggles to stay in school? How could your school make it easier for them to stay? Is there anything you could do in your classroom to make it easier for them? Could you get another child to help them with homework or to catch up when they have missed school?

Ideas for the classroom

Read the story of Martha to the children and let them discuss it, in groups. How would staying in school have helped Martha stay safe from HIV infection? How can school help anyone to stay safe from HIV?

It is also important to encourage children to discuss problems they have at home with a teacher before they feel that they need to drop out. Here are some questions that the class can discuss in groups.

- What can I do to make sure that I do not drop out of school?
- How can I encourage other children not to drop out?

Helpful hints

- To make your classroom more girl-friendly, look at your own attitudes to girls, and make sure that you encourage them as much as you do the boys. It is important that girls have good female role models to follow. Does your school respect female teachers as much as males? Are women given leadership roles?
- Check that girls don't have to do more chores than boys. Also check that girls are just as active during your lessons as the boys. Check that you do not let boys dominate the classroom discussions. Sometimes, put boys and girls into separate groups. Try to assist girls who are having trouble with menstruation, so that they don't miss school.

19 What puts children at risk of getting infected with HIV?

Definition

Being **at risk** – someone who can easily get HIV.

Identifying risks

The first step in helping young people to stay healthy and safe is to find out what puts them at risk. Because HIV is mainly transmitted through sex, we often think that young children will not get it easily – but some younger children might have got the virus from their mothers. Some children are already sexually active at the age of 13, or are at risk because they have been sexually abused.

Activity   Thinking about risks

It is very useful if the entire staff of your school does this exercise, so that you can see what needs special attention.

- What can you do to help reduce the risk to the children in your class?
- What can the school do to help keep the children safe from being infected with HIV?
- Are there any risks that you could add to the list of risks in the table?
- Which risks are the strongest among the children in your class?
- Which risks are the strongest among the people in your community?

What puts younger children at most risk?

Social problems	Behaviour	Lack of knowledge
There is possible sexual or emotional abuse. The family is poor. There are family problems. There is alcohol abuse in the family. The child is neglected. The child is an orphan – orphans are at special risk because they do not have the protection of the family. Children share rooms with adults, so they may have seen or heard sex.	Does not have skill to say 'NO' to sexual advances. Does not have skill to deal with peer pressure to become sexually active. Does not have high self-esteem and could use sex to make him/herself feel better. Does not have skill and understanding to stay with one sexual partner. May, like many children, be very curious and lack supervision.	Could be trying out sex without good information about how to protect themselves from HIV. Probably does not know everything about sex and sexual feelings. Probably does not believe that she or he is at risk because we cannot see if someone is HIV positive. Some parents do not talk to their children about sex, or they talk about it when it is already too late.

Ideas for the classroom

Try a 'traffic light' game to help children become aware of risky behaviour. You can make up your own stories that show risky behaviour. Each pupil colours in three cards – red, green and yellow. These show how much risk there is in the story of getting HIV.

Green: The situation is healthy and safe.

Red: Stop and run away, the situation is dangerous.

Yellow: Something is not right. Be careful. You are at risk.

Now tell the children stories, such as the three examples on page 41.

Preventing the spread of HIV and AIDS

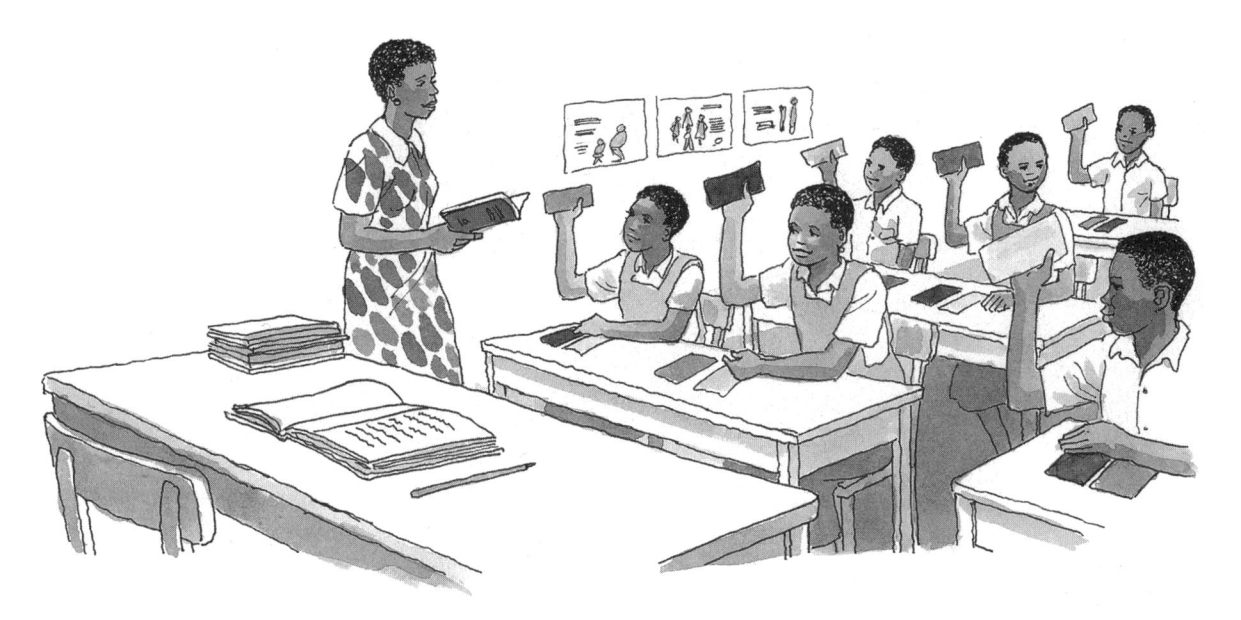

Helpful hints

Staff at your school need to think about what they can do if they find out that children are at risk as a result of social problems. Some ideas for the school could be:

- Make a list of all the services that are available in your community to deal with social problems.
- Keep a copy of this list in a place where every member of staff and children can have access to it.
- Let the children know who they can approach at the school if they feel they are at risk.

The children raise a card according how they see the level of risk. In their groups, the children give reasons why they chose their card.

Story 1
John is struggling with Mathematics. His teacher has offered to help him with his homework. John must come in the morning so that they will not be disturbed by anybody. When John gets there, the teacher gives him tea and cake and asks him into the bedroom to help make the bed.

Story 2
Every evening, Mary fetches water from the river. She often meets Ben there. She likes him. He is very handsome and sweet to her. He helps her to lift the heavy bucket onto her head. One evening, when no-one was around, he said he would carry her bucket if she gave him a kiss. He held her close and Mary felt very happy.

Story 3
Paulina is very sad. Her big brother has come back from the city because he is dying of AIDS. She really loves him. Every afternoon when she comes home from school she helps to bath him and to feed him. At night she tells him stories about her day. At weekends, she washes his clothes and sheets.

Stories can help children to understand how complicated and confusing the world can sometimes be. Once they have played the 'traffic light' game you could ask them to sit in their groups and make up more green stories, yellow stories and red stories. This will give you the chance to see how well they understand what can put them at risk.

20 Sexual abuse

Definitions

Sexual abuse is when an adult or a child does one of the following things:

- Shows a child his or her private parts.
- Touches a child's private parts, for example, with their hands, mouth or their own private parts.
- Shows pictures or movies to a child that are very sexy, or takes pictures of a child's private parts.
- Masturbates in front of a child, or forces the child to masturbate.

Rape is when the person is forced to have sexual intercourse.

Sexual harassment is if one person constantly touches another, asks for sexual favours or talks sexy, and if this makes the other person feel uncomfortable.

Helpful hints

- When teaching about abuse, it is very important to be sensitive and watch the children's responses carefully. If you suspect that a child in your class is being abused, you could encourage them to speak to someone they trust.
- Children also need to know that sexual abuse can cause them to be infected with HIV and that it is, therefore, very important to speak to someone they trust. Useful questions to help the child talk could be: 'Is someone making you unhappy?' 'Are you afraid of something?' 'Have you got a problem at home or at school?' 'Do you have someone to speak to?'
- It is also important to find out whether there is anybody in your community to whom a child could speak about rape or sexual abuse.

Children can be exposed to many dangerous situations where older children or adults want to force them to have sex or touch them in ways that are uncomfortable.

Teaching children to handle danger

From an early age, children need to be taught what sexual abuse is and about good and bad touching (see Topic 21, pages 44–45).

They also need to be given the skills to be assertive (see Topic 28, pages 60–61) and to say 'NO!' (See Topic 21, page 45)

Younger children may not need to know about the details of sexual abuse, but it is important that teachers have this information.

Signs of abuse

You may recognise a child who is being abused. For example:

- There may be a sudden change in behaviour that can't be explained.
- The child may be depressed or suicidal.
- The child may burst into tears easily.
- The child may suddenly be withdrawn.
- The child may want lots of attention.
- The child may not be able to concentrate.
- The child may lie or steal.
- The child may not trust adults.

Ideas for the classroom

Most types of sexual abuse happen with people that the children know. That is why it is very important that children know what to do. The pictures opposite show some dangerous situations children can find themselves in. Tell them the stories and let them discuss, or even act out, what the victim could do next to stay safe.

Preventing the spread of HIV and AIDS

If you don't co-operate, I'm going tell your mother what a bad girl you really are.

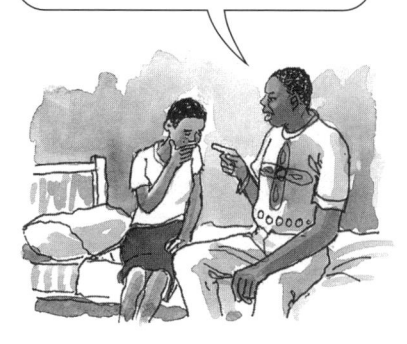

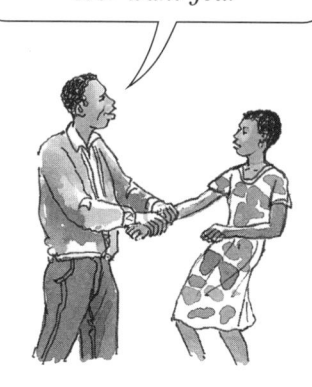

Threats

If you two pretty girls come with me, I'll give you a very nice present.

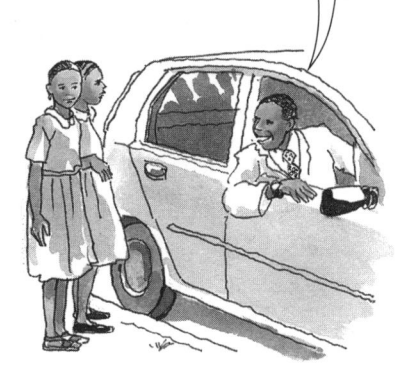

Gifts

Don't refuse me, young girl. You're so ugly. No one will ever want you.

Humiliation

Please come in here and help me close my zip.

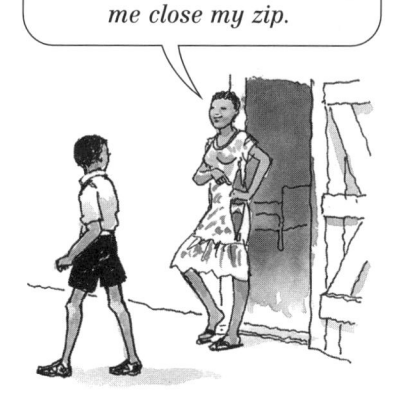

Being tricked

This is our little secret. You don't have to tell anyone, do you?

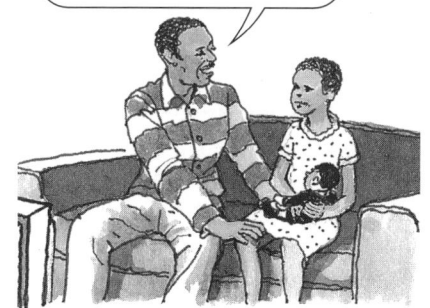

More tricks

You'll do what I say, or else I'll …

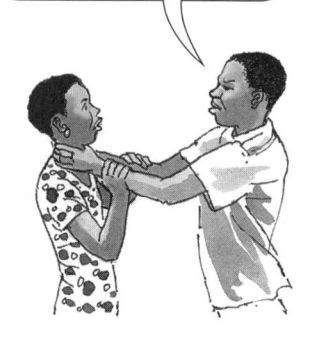

Violence

Activity Find out about the law and school policy

- Many countries have different laws about sexual abuse. Find out what the laws of your country are.
- At what age are people allowed to have sex?
- Are there any laws against sexual harassment in your country?
- Have any of the pupils at your school been abused? How does your school deal with it?
- Does your school have a policy against sexual harassment?
- Find out about the organisations in your country that help children who have been/are being abused. Let your pupils know about these organisations, what their names are and how they can be contacted.

21 Helping young children to stay safe from abuse

Recognising unacceptable behaviour

It is very important that younger children are taught to recognise what feels uncomfortable and for them to have the confidence to say so. Often it is not clear to children, especially very young ones, whether what is happening to them is acceptable or unacceptable.

Ideas for the classroom

Teach the children about good touching, bad touching and confusing touching.

- Good touching feels like something is being given or shared with you. Examples are: hugs, mother stroking your hair, holding hands. Ask: 'Can you think of other types of good touching? How do you feel when a touch is good? What do you do when a touch is good?'
- Bad touching feels uncomfortable, as if someone is taking something away from you. This can be when someone touches your buttocks or private parts without your permission. Or someone hits, pushes or holds you too tight. Sometimes tickling or wrestling can be bad touching, if it does not stop. Ask: 'Can you think of other types of bad touching? How do you feel when a touch is bad? What do you do when a touch is bad?'
- Confusing touching is when the touch is not clearly good or bad. Hugs, kisses, slapping and pinching can all be confusing. It is when we don't know what the person means by it, when the person says something that does not fit with the touch.

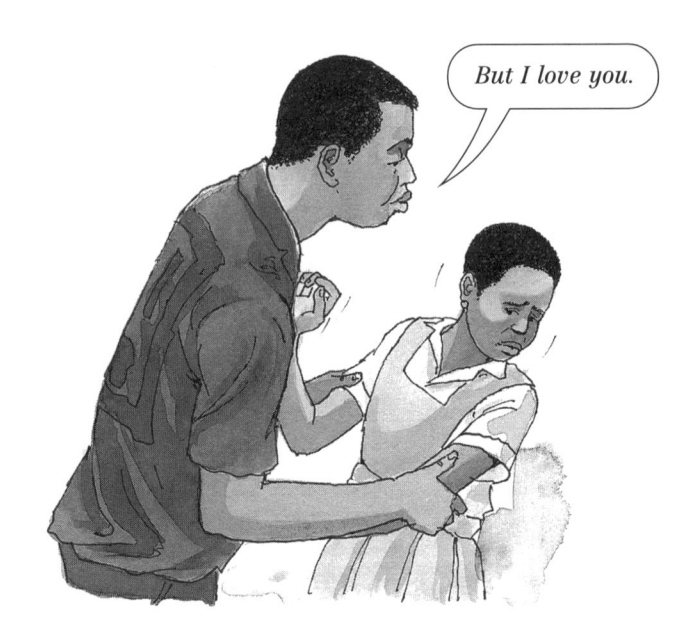

But I love you.

Preventing the spread of HIV and AIDS

Ask, 'Can you think of other types of confusing touching? How do you feel when a touch is confusing? What do you do when a touch is confusing?'

Teach children these rules about what to do if someone touches them in a way that feels bad or confusing. Afterwards, you could put them up on the wall:

> If someone touches me badly:
> - I will ask them to stop.
> - I will say that I will tell someone.
> - I will run away if I can.
> - I can shout for help.
> - I mustn't fight, unless I know that I am stronger than the other person.
> - I can tell someone I trust, such as a parent, teacher or guardian, what happened.

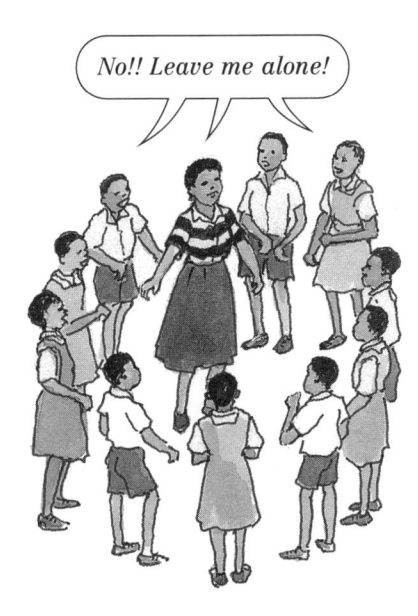

No!! Leave me alone!

Practise saying 'NO!'

It is important to practise with the children how to say 'NO!' in a dangerous or uncomfortable situation. This is especially important for very young children, who might feel ashamed to speak rudely to an adult.

Let children stand in a circle. The teacher or one of the children stands in the middle and says something that makes the child uncomfortable. For example: 'Come, my little child, here are some sweets.' 'Come here, and I'll kiss you.'

All the children shout as loudly as they can: 'NO! I don't want sweets.' Or, 'NO! Leave me alone!'

Let them repeat it and then let each child shout it alone. If their voices are soft, let them practise until they sound fierce.

Helpful hints

Let the children learn these rules by heart. You could translate them into the mother tongue for them.

1. My body is my own.
2. I have the right to decide who touches me, how they touch me and when.
3. No one should look at or touch my private parts in a way that makes me uncomfortable.
4. I can trust my feelings about what feels right and what does not feel right.

22 Changing the way we behave

Definition

The **age of consent** is the legal age from when people are allowed to have sexual intercourse. Each country decides on this age. Some countries have decided that 16 is the age of consent, others have chosen 18. Some countries have a different age of consent for men and women.

Did you know?

Marriage is not always safe. Early marriage, marriage to a person who already has had many partners, or to someone who is unfaithful, marriage to a man who already has a wife (polygamy) and marriage without testing for HIV may not be safe.

Steps towards keeping children safe

The first step towards keep our children safe and healthy is by supporting them in safe behaviours, such as abstaining from sex. The second step is to change any behaviour that is risky to safe behaviour. We need to persuade children to delay having sex until they are ready to get married. Marriage or sexual relationships should always be after the age of consent.

Once they decide that they are ready, both partners need to be tested and discuss how they are going to stay safe. It is important to stay faithful to one partner and to use condoms.

Change is difficult

But changing the way we behave is very difficult. This is why it is very important that safe behaviour is supported by teachers, peers and the community.

Changing sexual behaviour is often even more difficult than changing behaviour in other areas of our lives. This is because there is much confusion and silence around sex. To change sexual behaviour, children need support from many sides. Research now suggests that it is possible for some young people who have started sex to stop, but they need motivation and support. Those children who are not sexually active need to be supported in this and given skills to stay safe in future. These skills include recognising risky situations, being assertive and resisting pressure from peers or adults.

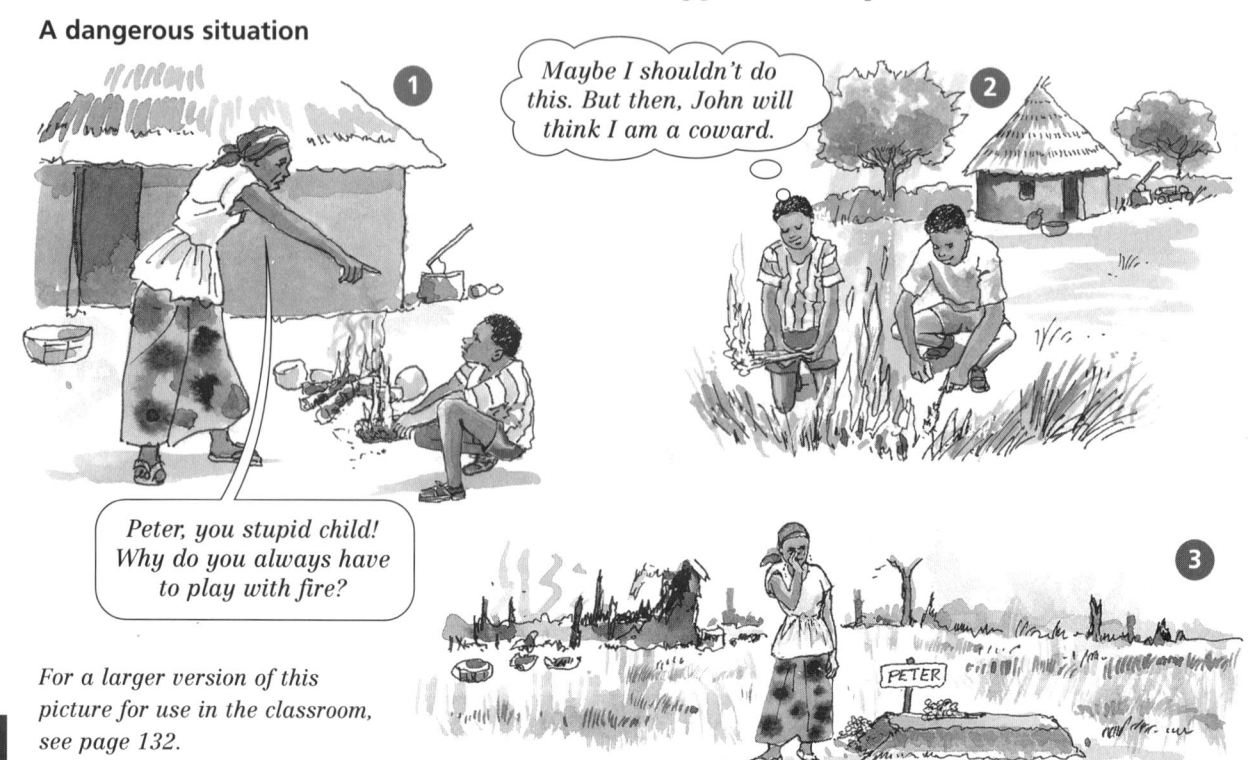

A dangerous situation

For a larger version of this picture for use in the classroom, see page 132.

Preventing the spread of HIV and AIDS

Activity Thinking about changing behaviour

Think of some behaviour you have tried to change. Maybe you have wanted to stop smoking or drinking, maybe you have wanted to save money, lose weight or get fit.

- How did you try to change?
- What three things helped you?
- What three things made it more difficult?

How to change behaviour

To change behaviour we need to:

- know that what we are doing is risky
- want to change for positive reasons (e.g. so that we can benefit in future)
- choose to change our behaviour
- get new skills and knowledge
- be supported and motivated to change
- try out our new knowledge and skills
- be successful in our new behaviour.

Discussing the story of Peter

The story of Peter shows how difficult it can be to change dangerous behaviour. With the class, look at the story and discuss it.

- Why do you think the boys did something as dangerous as playing with fire?
- Do you think they really knew, or believed, that it could kill them?
- Why do you think Peter did not listen to his mother?
- Do you think he wanted to impress his friend?
- Do you think he would have played with fire if he could have looked into the future?

Here are some ideas that could have helped to change Peter's risky behaviour.

- His mother could have motivated him better by speaking clearly and calmly to him.
- Peter knew that what he was doing was wrong. He needed the skill to stand up for what he knew.

What advice would you add to this?

Ideas for the classroom

Use the pictures of Peter and his friend to talk to children about changing risky behaviour. Ask about why they think Peter and his friend played with fire. Also talk about how Peter could have been helped to change his behaviour and stay safe. Link the story to a discussion of how we sometimes do things that are not safe. Ask, 'Why do we sometimes do things that we have been told not to do?' Remind children how difficult it is to change our behaviour.

In groups, let pupils discuss what could put them at risk of getting infected with HIV. Let them find ways in which they can change their behaviour to stay safe. They can then report back to the whole class.

Helpful hints

When trying to change the behaviour of your pupils, remember the following points.

- Don't preach.
- Be patient. As you know yourself, changing behaviour takes time and persistence.
- Always ask for help if you feel that you can't cope alone with trying to help the children in your care.

23 Helping children to make positive choices

Definition
Self-esteem is having a good opinion of yourself.

Did you know?
Sometimes, adults are afraid that a child with high self-esteem will become disrespectful and cheeky. This is not true. Bad behaviour often comes from low self-esteem. Such a child needs to show off. High self-esteem allows a child to calm down and get on with the job.

The difficulties young people face

Being young can be a difficult time, especially when there are problems in the family, such as poverty or bad relationships. As children become adults, life can be very confusing.

From being quite carefree and confident, children suddenly start to worry about what others think about them – they wonder whether they are attractive enough, clever enough, strong enough, etc.

Some children suffer from hopelessness and depression. They worry about their future. Children can also feel very lonely. They feel that adults do not understand them. Some young children have sex to make them feel better about themselves, or for gifts, or because of abuse. This makes them very vulnerable to getting infected with HIV.

To help children make positive choices it is important to build their self-esteem from early in primary school, and to help them set goals for the future.

Ideas for the classroom

Set goals for the future

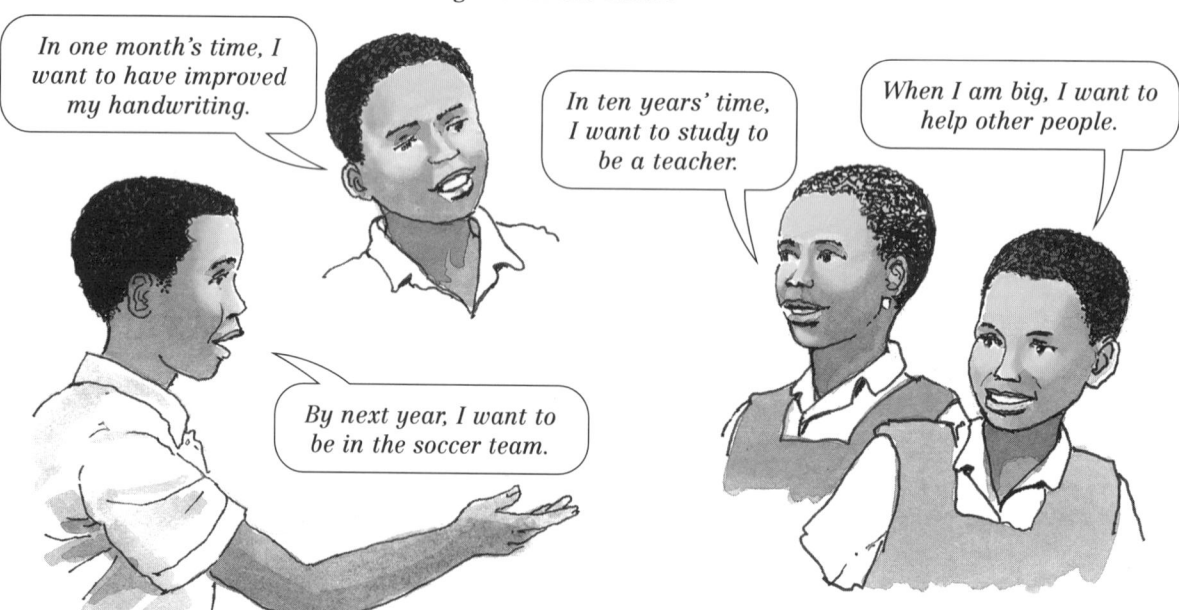

In one month's time, I want to have improved my handwriting.

In ten years' time, I want to study to be a teacher.

When I am big, I want to help other people.

By next year, I want to be in the soccer team.

Children can make positive choices about their health and staying safe if they feel that they have a purpose in life.

Help children to find out what their dreams for the future are. Some will know the answer immediately while others struggle. You can help those who struggle by asking them to think of a person they admire. Let the children complete the sentences in the box. Encourage them not to limit their dreams.

Preventing the spread of HIV and AIDS

- In <u>one year</u> from today, I want to achieve ………
- In <u>five years</u> from today, I want to achieve ………
- In <u>ten years</u> from today, I want to achieve ………

Now ask learners to think of some short-term goals they can achieve by next week or next month that will help them reach these dreams.

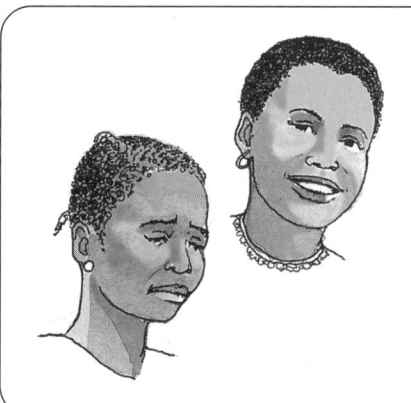

Case study

Here is the story of two girls.

Mavis and Grace are 15 years old. But they respond to life very differently.

Grace seems to be happy much of the time. When she gets bad marks in school, she just tries to work harder. Last year, her boyfriend left her and she cried a lot. But then she decided that it was probably better that he left. When she feels very stressed, she goes for a long walk next to the river. She also likes to speak to her best friend about her problems.

When Mavis fails a test, she blames the teacher. When she gets stressed, she likes to go to the bar and speak to men and drink beer. When her boyfriend left her, she was very depressed and said bad things about him to everybody.

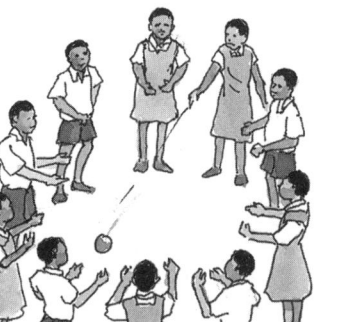

Build self-esteem

Discuss Grace and Mavis. Building your pupils' self-esteem can take a lot of patience and time. It is a very important part of keeping young people safe because it helps them to resist peer pressure.

Let the children stand in a circle. One child starts by throwing a ball to another one. The one who catches has to say something good about the thrower, for example, 'You are kind.' 'You are clever.' 'You can read well.' 'You know how to ride a bicycle.' 'Your hair is pretty.'

Grace has much more self-esteem than Mavis.

- How can we see this?
- What do you think can build self-esteem? What is the difference between having good self-esteem and being arrogant?
- How does self-esteem get destroyed?
- How do you think Mavis' teacher could help her to improve her self-esteem?

Helpful hints

Affirm the children in your classroom.

- Listen carefully to what they say and take time to answer their questions.
- Praise them when they have achieved something. This should be done not only with academic achievements but also for positive behaviour, like being kind or having tried to do something that is difficult.
- Encourage them to be realistic about situations. If, for example, a child struggles, she or he may say or feel: 'I am stupid.' You could say: 'You are not stupid, maybe you should just spend a bit more time on Maths.'
- Be constructive when you criticise. You can reject bad behaviour ('What you did is wrong') but not the person ('You are a bad and stupid boy!').

24 The ABCD of prevention

The ABCD of prevention

- Children need to know that **abstaining** from sex is the safest choice.
- If it is not possible to abstain, the next best thing is to **be faithful** to one partner for life, after testing for HIV.
- If someone is having sex, it is best to use a **condom** to protect both partners.
- Staying healthy and free from sexually transmitted **disease** is also part of protecting yourself from getting infected with HIV. People with STDs get HIV more easily and pass it on more easily.

What is the 'ABCD of Prevention'?

The main reason for the spread of HIV is that people have unprotected sex. This includes children.

The *ABCD of Prevention* is a slogan that is used in many countries to prevent the spread of HIV and AIDS. It stands for the choices we make to stay safe: **A**bstain, **B**e faithful, **C**ondomise and stay free from sexually transmitted **D**isease.

Even if children are not sexually active, it is very important that they are taught about the *ABCD of Prevention*. This is so that they can be safe when they get older and, also, so that they can pass on the information to others.

To stay safe and to pass on correct information, it is very important that children have all the information about prevention from an early age. This includes information about condoms and how they are used.

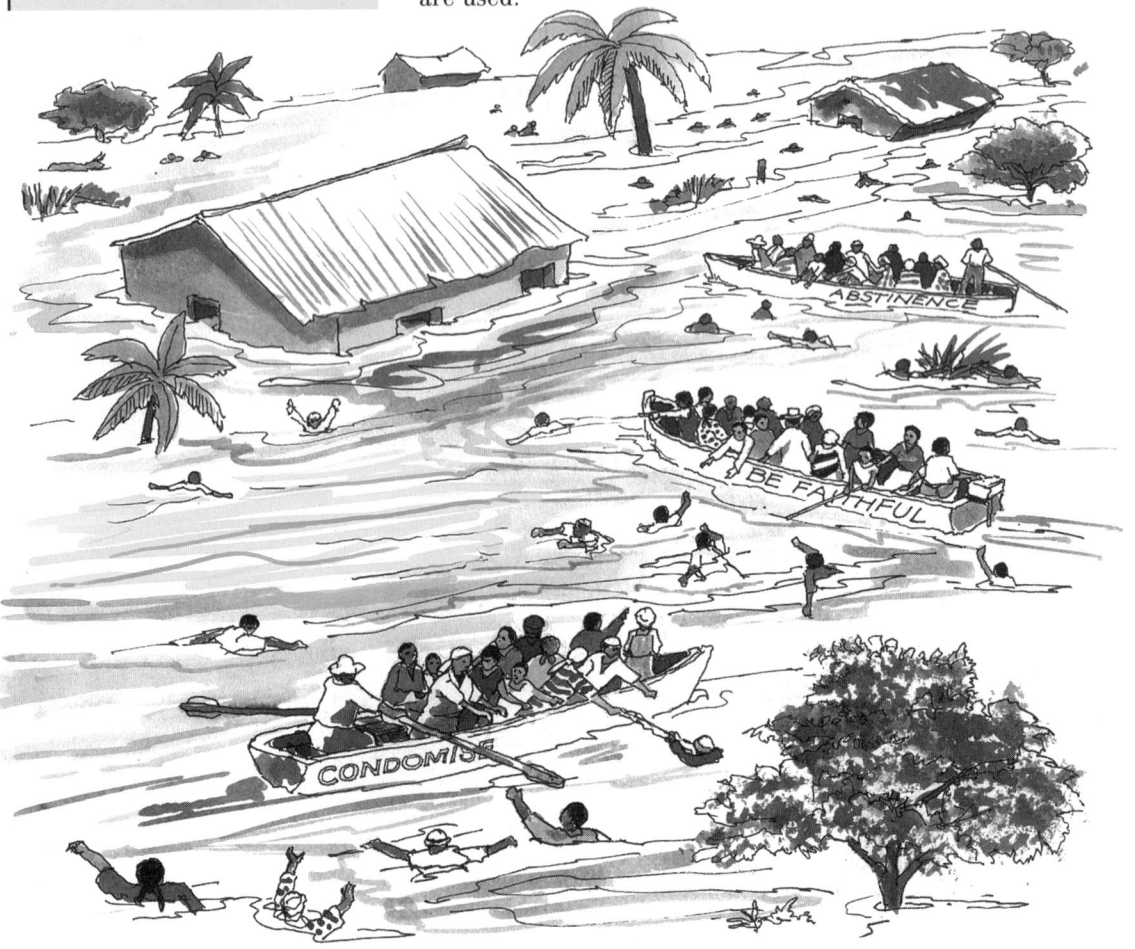

The ideas on this page come from materials produced by Fr Bernard Joinet for the *The Fleet of Hope* resources, produced jointly with the Tanzania AIDS project.

Preventing the spread of HIV and AIDS

Did you know?

Many people today prefer to use the term 'Sexually Transmitted Infections' (STIs) rather than 'Sexually Transmitted Diseases'. Both terms are correct, and mean the same thing. In this book, we use 'Diseases' so that we can talk about the 'ABCD' of prevention – which is easy to remember.

Ideas for the classroom

Tell children that HIV and AIDS are like a flood that can kill many people. Luckily there are some boats that one can climb onto to stay safe. These boats are *ABSTAIN, BE FAITHFUL* and *CONDOMISE*. Use the picture opposite in your classroom to introduce the ABC of prevention. Adapt the questions to the level of the children. Remember that the idea is not to look for the right answers but to get children to think about preventing HIV and AIDS. Explain that it is also important to stay free of sexually transmitted disease (the 'D' of prevention).

Encourage the children to be creative and find other ways to illustrate the ABCD of prevention. Ask children to make a poster which will teach others about the ABCD of prevention. Have a competition for the group that can come up with the most creative idea to persuade people to stay safe. You could put up these posters in the school.

Discussing the picture

Discuss the following questions with your colleagues and friends. They will help you to think about the ABC of prevention. You can check some of your ideas on the next few pages where the ABCD is discussed. Look at the picture on the opposite page.

- Why do you think the people have chosen the boat they are in to stay safe from the flood?
- Which boat do you think is the safest?
- How can one help people get into a safer boat without falling into the water?
- Do you think people could fall out of the boat still? Why?
- How can one help the people who are in the water get into a boat?

Helpful hints

Before you teach about the ABCD of prevention it is important to find out what children already know about the topic. Especially with a difficult topic such as this, it is important that you understand the level your pupils are at. If you speak about things they do not understand or which they already know about, children will often misbehave or switch off. This can make it difficult to teach about HIV and AIDS.

25 The A of prevention – Abstaining

Remember

Research shows that sex education and information about condoms **do not** encourage young people to have sex earlier. Providing accurate information about sex encourages young people to delay having sex and take actions to protect themselves.

Teaching about abstaining

The message to abstain from sex is the most important, especially for children. It can also be the most difficult because there are many things that encourage young people, including children, to have sex.

It does not help just to tell young people that they must abstain – they need lots of ongoing support and many skills. Topics 28 and 30 (pages 60–61 and 64–65), deal with the skills of assertiveness and resisting peer pressure, which can help young people to abstain.

Decisions about having sex are often made in a hurry or under the influence of alcohol. One way to help children to abstain is to make them think about having sex when they are calm – before they are under pressure. You can also help them to avoid alcohol.

Ideas for the classroom

Why do we have sex?

Ask the children to look at this list of why some young people decide to have sex. Here are some common reasons.

- Because they are attracted to someone, or believe they are in love.
- To please the other person.
- To prove love to each other.
- They are afraid that the relationship will break up without sex.
- They are curious to see what it is all about.
- They are afraid of being mocked or beaten.
- They are offered money or presents.

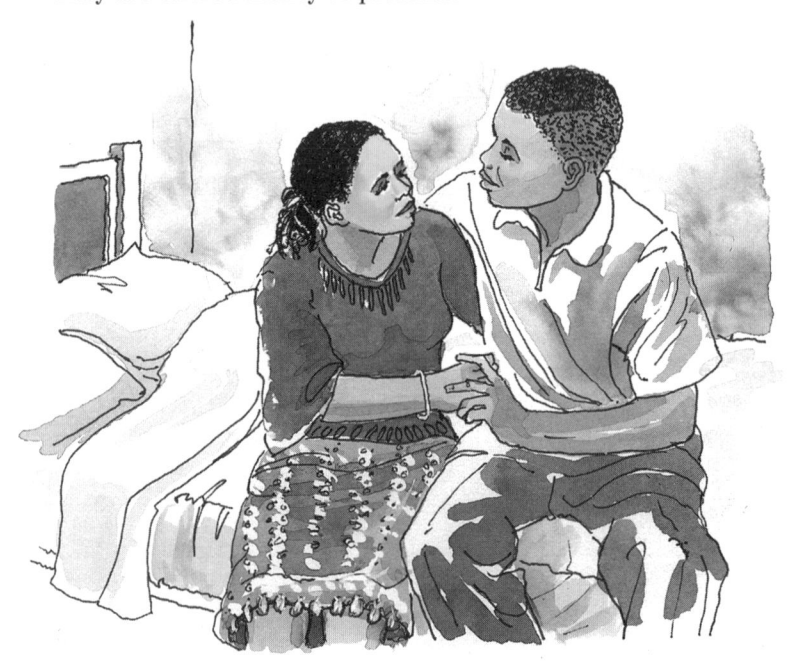

Young people may decide to have sex for many different reasons.

Preventing the spread of HIV and AIDS

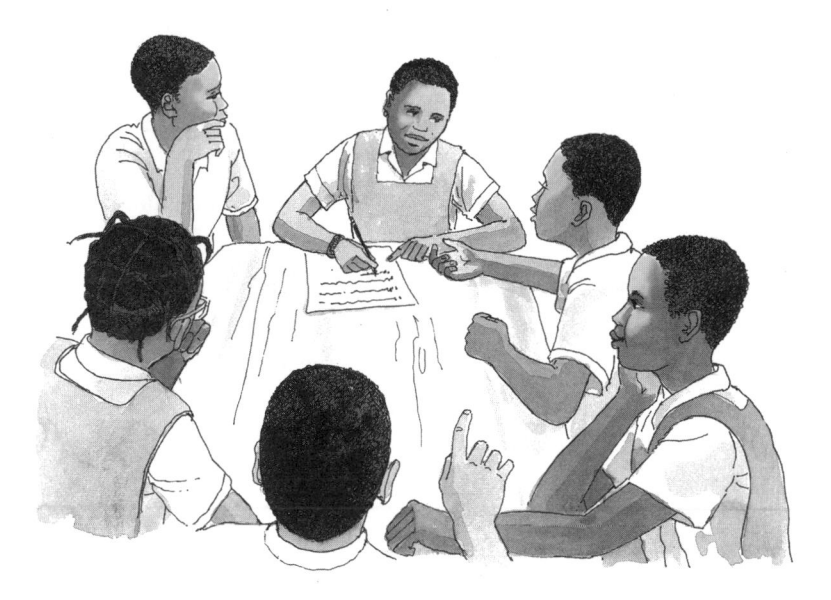

- They want to help their families survive or continue in school.
- They want affection and love.
- They get carried away by strong sexual feelings.
- They are looking for excitement.
- They believe that everybody else is having sex and they want to be like everybody else.

Ask them to discuss which of these reasons are good reasons, and which ones are poor.

In groups, let the children add more reasons of their own.

Why do we abstain?

Talk to the children about these reasons why some young people are delaying having sex.

- They want to get an education and not get pregnant too early.
- They want to wait to have sex till they meet a really special person.
- They are afraid of getting HIV.
- They don't feel they are with the right person.
- They don't feel that they want to have sex yet.
- It goes against their religious values.
- They are worried that the person they have sex with will no longer respect them and will leave them.

Ask them to add more of their own ideas.

Teaching about HIV and AIDS

How can we abstain?

The following is a good exercise to start talking about healthy relationships between males and females. Sexual relationships and issues of pregnancy are looked at in greater detail in Section 4.

Ask pupils to name four things that could help a person to abstain from sex.

Here is some more advice on how to abstain.

- Don't go out with people who you don't trust.
- Always go to parties and events with your friends.
- Before you go out with another person, decide how far you are prepared to go with this person. Will you let them kiss you? Hug you? Touch your private parts? What will you do if they do something you don't want?
- From the beginning, make it clear to the person that you don't want to have sex yet.
- Listen to your feelings. When you feel uncomfortable, leave.
- Avoid going to someone's house when there is no one else there.
- Don't accept favours, presents, money or lifts from anybody you don't know very well, and who you do not trust.
- Even if you know a person well, when they give you a present and you feel uncomfortable, think about, or even ask them, what they expect from you if you take the gift. You can refuse to accept it or give it back later.
- Show gifts you have received to your parents or someone you trust and tell them who gave them to you.

A myth

Some people believe that if you do not have sex you will be sick and your penis will shrivel or your breasts won't grow. This is not true. Abstinence is healthy. You do not need to have sex to grow or be strong.

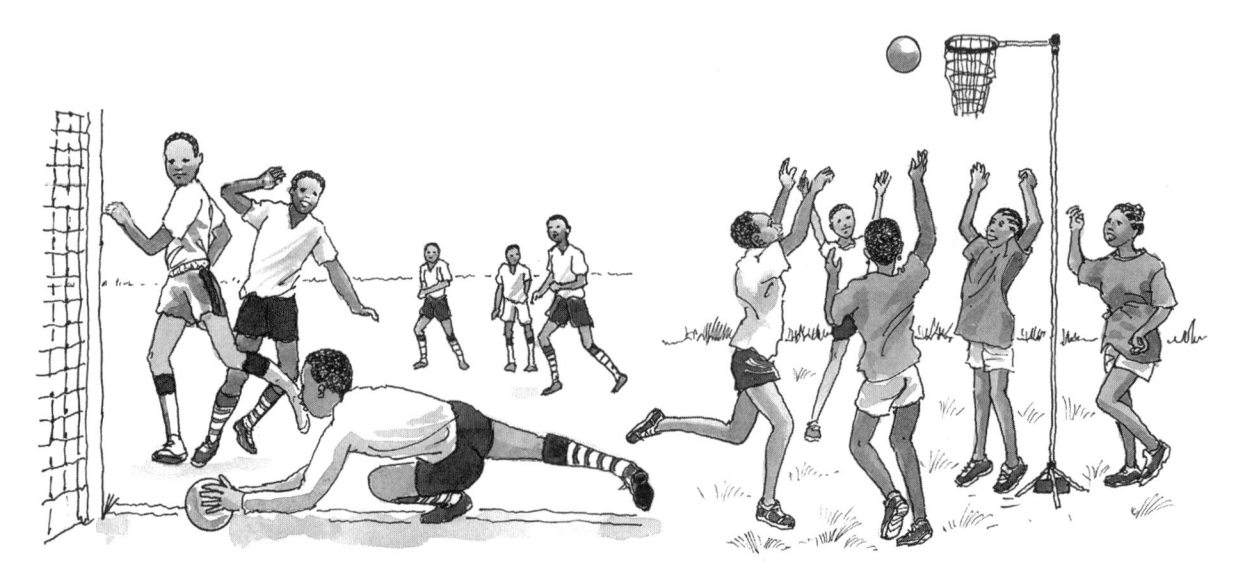

Getting involved in activities, such as sport, can help young people abstain from sex.

Preventing the spread of HIV and AIDS

- Avoid alcohol.
- Get involved in positive activities such as sport, hobbies and youth clubs.

How can we show affection without having sex?

Young people need to know that they can have boy-girl relationships without having sex. They also need to know that once they have had sex, they can stop again.

To help them, discuss how people can show that they like each other without having sex. For example by holding hands, giving a flower, kissing, touching, writing a letter, hugging.

In groups, let children think of more ways in which they can show that they like each other.

26 The B of Prevention – Be faithful

Activity A discussion

Here are some questions to ask yourself as a teacher or to discuss in a group with your colleagues.

- Do I believe that it is really possible to be faithful in a relationship?
- Does my culture expect men to be faithful to one woman and women to be faithful to one man?
- Do we have the same rules of faithfulness for men as we have for women?
- How can I teach children about being faithful if my environment does not really promote it?
- How can I be a good role model for relationships?

Preparation for adult life

The message about being faithful is more for older people who are in relationships, especially when they are married. However, children need to be taught about this, to prepare them for adult life.

It is important to emphasise that **being faithful is only safe if both partners have taken an HIV test and are negative, and then remain faithful to each other for the rest of their lives.** Being faithful to one person for a while, and then to the next person, is not very safe. Also, we cannot always be certain our partner is being faithful – and relationships we want to last for ever may end. This is why it is always safest to use condoms even in a close relationship, such as marriage.

Although children generally don't form strong sexual partnerships, it is important that they start thinking about healthy and loving relationships from an early age. Children get most of their information about relationships from watching adults. Many of our societies do not really encourage faithfulness and allow different standards for men and for women. It is therefore very important that we, as adults, look at our own attitudes towards faithfulness and relationships.

Ideas for the classroom

Young people often fall in and out of love. They will develop a very powerful feeling for somebody, which goes away just as quickly as it started. This is called 'an infatuation.' It is important that they start looking at and understanding for themselves what kind of relationship feels healthy and respectful to them.

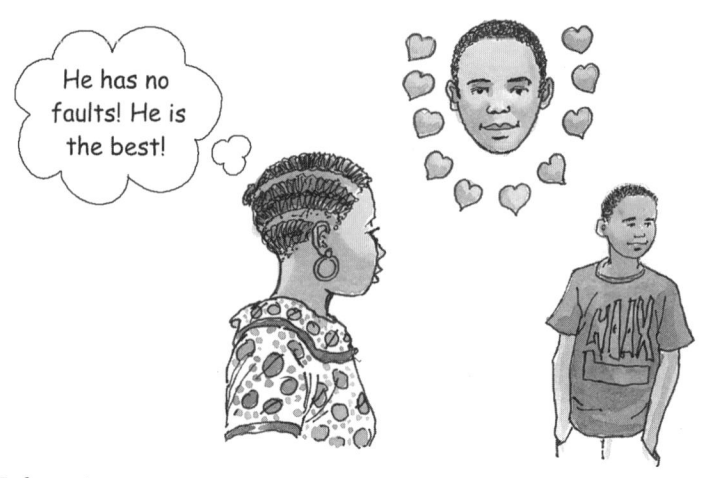

Infatuation

Preventing the spread of HIV and AIDS

Here is an exercise you can do with the children.

- Each child writes down what qualities they like in another person.
- Then they get into groups of girls and boys.

Each group discusses:

- What qualities or behaviour do you expect in a good and healthy friendship/relationship?
- How do you see if someone has these qualities or behaviours?

Here are some examples.

> I expect to be respected. Someone shows me respect when they listen to what I say.
>
> I expect to be treated with kindness. Someone is kind to me when they stop doing something that causes me pain.
>
> I expect someone to stand by me in difficult times. Someone does that by not believing bad things about me if people talk about me badly.

All the girls get together and decide what are the most important qualities and behaviour they want from a boyfriend. All the boys get together and decide what behaviour and qualities they would like from a girlfriend.

Bring the class together again and write down all the most important qualities in a friendship between boys and girls. Then let the class decide on the most important qualities.

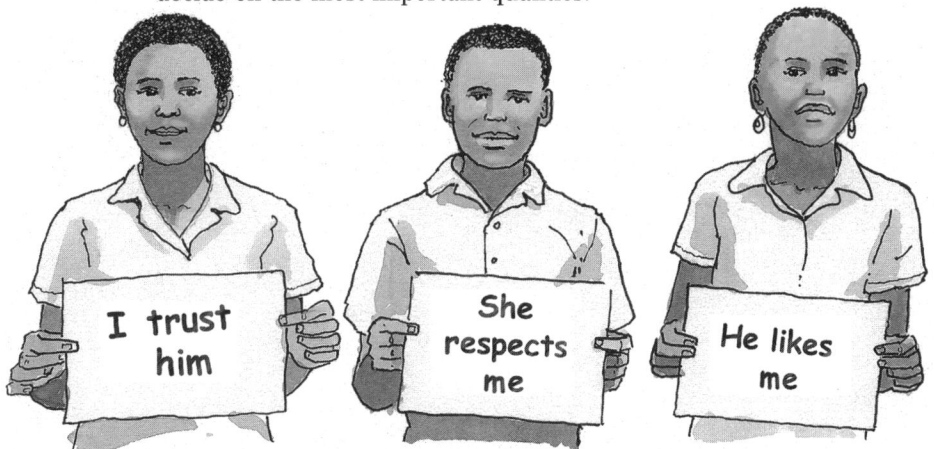

Discuss with children the words *loyalty* and *faithfulness*. Think about what they mean and ask children to find the words in their mother tongue. Discuss why loyalty and faithfulness are important in keeping oneself and one's partner safe.

If you feel that the children in your class are ready to discuss such issues, ask whether they think that married couples can always trust each other. Make sure that you emphasise that it is safest to wear condoms, as one never knows whether someone has been faithful.

27 The C of Prevention – Condomise

Remember

Teaching about condoms does **not** encourage children to try out sex. This is especially true if it is taught together with the message of abstinence.

Activity A discussion

With your colleagues and school management, discuss how you could prepare parents for the fact that you are going to teach about condoms. How would you explain why it is important to teach about condoms?

Learning about condoms

It is important that children, from an early age, know about condoms, so that they become comfortable and familiar with the idea of using them when they later come to have sex. We never know when they can get into a situation where a condom can save them from being infected with HIV. Remember, many children leave school at the end of their primary years, or drop out of school. We cannot leave teaching about condoms until secondary school.

When teaching about condoms it is important to tell children that:

- delaying sex is best for children (see Topic 25, page 52)
- most condoms don't fit boys in primary school. It is best for them to abstain from sex
- if they are used correctly, condoms can protect against HIV, other sexually transmitted diseases (STDs) and pregnancy (for information on STDs, see Topic 39, pages 84–85)
- condoms can slip or break, so they are not 100 per cent protection
- people should never have sex without a condom unless they have both tested for HIV, know they are both free from HIV and are ready to have sex and be faithful for life
- abstinence or delaying sex is best for children.

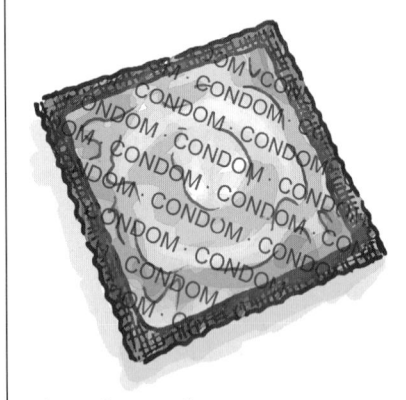

A condom packet

A condom

Important information about condoms

This is the information you need to answer questions that the children might have about condoms. If you don't know something, be honest and find out for them. See also Topic 6, page 14, which mentions myths about condoms.

You could also ask a local health worker to help with giving information about condoms.

What is a condom?

It is a soft rubber tube that is put on a man's penis before sex. It is to stop the semen containing sperm from coming into contact with the woman and to stop the fluids in her vagina from touching his penis. It can stop pregnancy and infection with HIV and other STDs.

Are condoms safe?

Very seldom, a condom can break. But, used correctly, they can help to protect us. A condom is much safer than no condom.

What can make a condom not safe?

- If the condom is old. There is a date on the packet that tells you whether you can still use it. An old one may break.

Preventing the spread of HIV and AIDS

Helpful hints

- Bringing condoms to school is a good way to teach about them but it may not be acceptable in your community. Check with your school principal or authorities.
- Teachers may be embarrassed to answer questions about condoms. Try to overcome this shyness and always be positive and factual about condoms.
- If your religion prevents you from informing children about condoms, talk more about abstinence and let another teacher or health worker teach your class about condoms.

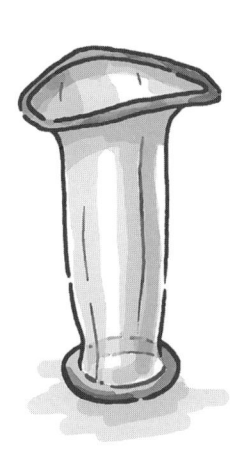

- If the packet is broken or damaged, or if you tear it when opening the packet.
- If a man uses two condoms with one on top of the other.
- If a condom is used more than once. It has to be thrown away immediately after it is used.
- If oil has touched the condom it can break. For example, cooking oil or Vaseline.
- If the condom has been left in a hot place for too long.
- If a woman's vagina is too dry, the condom can break.
- If the condom breaks when you put it on. You should never unroll the condom before putting it on.

Where do you get condoms?

Condoms can be bought from some shops, such as supermarkets and pharmacies, and clinics usually have condoms.

How do you use a condom?

Wait for the penis to go hard and the woman's vagina to be wet inside before you put the condom on.

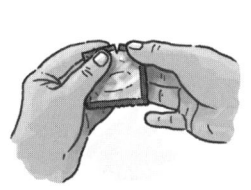

Open the packet on the side. Don't use your teeth or nails.

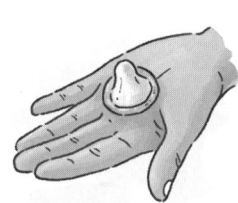

Put the condom on your hand with one side up, like a hat.

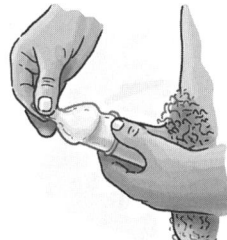

Pinch the end of the condom to squeeze out the air. Put the condom on the end of the penis and unroll it all the way down.

When the male has released his sperm (ejaculated), he should pull out the penis when it is still hard. He should hold the condom on the penis as he does this.

Take the condom off and tie a knot in it to stop the semen escaping. Throw the condom in a pit latrine, bury it, or burn it. Make sure children can't play with it.

There are also female condoms. These prevent sperm from coming into contact with the vagina. They work almost like a male condom, but a woman puts it into her vagina. They are made from strong material and, like a male condom, can only be used once.

Ideas for the classroom

Maybe you can prepare the lesson with some colleagues to help you become more comfortable.

You can demonstrate on a broomstick or on a potato how a condom is used.

Welcome all questions. Remember that there is no such thing as a stupid question.

You may want to separate boys and girls when you teach about condoms. It will make each group feel freer to ask questions.

28 Assertiveness skills

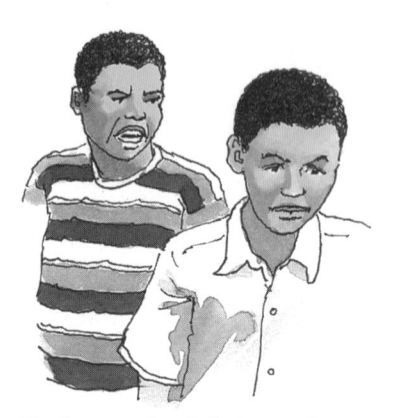

The boy on the right is passive.

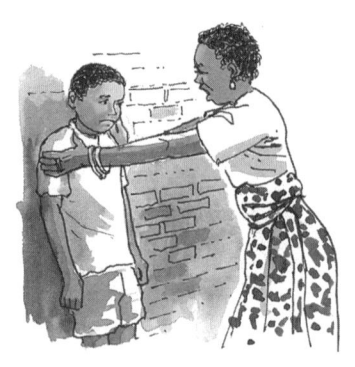

The woman is being aggressive.

What is assertiveness?

Being assertive is the most important skill to help young people stay safe.

Being **assertive** means standing up for yourself. It means being honest with yourself and other people about what you need and what feels comfortable. A person who is assertive will know when they feel ready for sex and be able to say so. A person who is assertive can also insist on using a condom.

People who are **passive** don't do anything to stand up for their rights. Even when they are treated badly, they don't do anything to protect their feelings or bodies from being hurt. They keep quiet when they are unhappy about something. They always put other people's needs before their own.

Being **aggressive** means putting your needs above anybody else's, even if other people suffer. Aggressive people are often rude or unkind. They force other people to do things they don't want to do. People who are aggressive may force others to have sex with them and to obey them.

In many cultures women and children are expected to be passive while boys and men are taught to be aggressive. Girls are taught to be passive towards boys. These attitudes can be dangerous, because women and children often cannot protect themselves from unsafe sex. A woman might find it difficult to insist that her partner uses a condom, and a child might find it difficult to avoid abuse.

Activity Think about assertiveness

- Is assertiveness encouraged in your community and in your school? Are boys stopped when they are aggressive? Are girls encouraged to be assertive?
- Think about the last time you were aggressive. What happened? How did it make you feel?
- Think about the last time you were passive. What happened? How did it make you feel?
- Think about the last time you were assertive. What happened? How did it make you feel? Why do you think you felt good about yourself?
- Explain the difference between these behaviours to your friends and exchange stories.

Ideas for the classroom

It is very important that children recognise the difference between aggressive, passive and assertive behaviour. Explain the words to them and ask them to find words in their own language that are like the word 'assertive'.

Assertiveness tips

Here are some tips to help you, as a teacher, to be more assertive, and to pass that on to your pupils.

- When you feel uncertain or pushed, give yourself time to decide what you feel or want.
- Say what you feel clearly. If the other person does not want to hear you, say it again.
- Keep eye contact. It tells the other person that you are serious.
- Don't apologise for how you feel or what you want.
- Don't get confused by the other person's argument. Just repeat what you want or don't want.
- Listen to the other person. Don't condemn them, just listen.

Preventing the spread of HIV and AIDS

Three scenarios

Let children act out these three different scenarios and identify how Susan is behaving. Explain that Fred and Susan have been together for two years. Fred feels that it is time for them to have sex. Here are three ways that Susan can react.

Discuss why being assertive is the best way to handle the situation.

Scenario 1

Fred: I think we have been together long enough now. I want to have sex with you.
Susan does not want to. She looks away and sinks into herself.
Fred: What do you think Susan?
Susan: I don't know.
Fred: Come on Susan, you know I love you.
Susan (reluctantly): I suppose. If you say so.

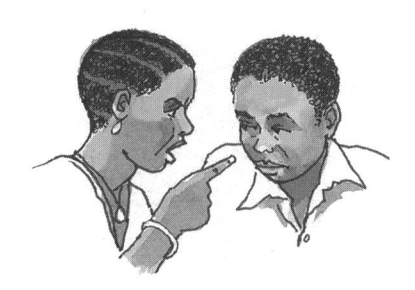

Scenario 2

Fred: I think we have been together long enough now. I want to have sex with you.
Susan (standing very close to Fred and shouting): How dare you ask such a thing? You dirty boy!
Fred: But I just thought …
Susan (interrupting him, shouting): All you can think about is sex!

Scenario 3

Fred: I think we have been together long enough now. I want to have sex with you.
Susan (calmly, looking him in the eyes): I really like you, but I'm not ready yet.
Fred: Oh come on Susan, we have been going out for so long I am sure you are ready.
Susan (staying calm): I know that I am not ready yet, Fred.
Fred: Come on Susan, don't you love me?
Susan: Yes I do, but I am not ready yet, Fred.
Fred: But if you really loved me, you would.
Susan: I am not ready, Fred. *(She walks away.)*

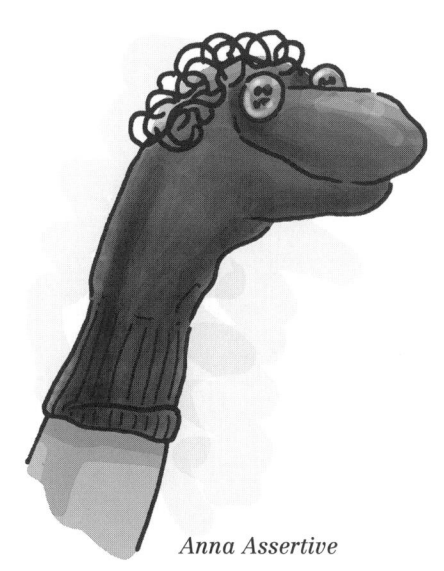

Anna Assertive

Make a puppet of Anna Assertive out of an old sock and allow children to speak through her. Encourage children to think about what Anna Assertive would do in many familiar situations, for example, if someone is being bullied or pushed. Using a puppet will also make it easier to practise being assertive with adults.

For example, ask Anna Assertive to stop doing her class-work and go and hit another child. Pretend to be really angry if Anna refuses. You can say something like: 'You have to listen to me, I am your teacher.' Or 'If you don't listen I will hit you.'

Afterwards, talk to the children about the experience. Speak about when we have to be assertive and what is the difference between being cheeky and being assertive.

Children need to know that, in the beginning, it is difficult to be assertive but, the more they practise, the easier it gets. All the time, refer back to the tips on how to be more assertive. You can make up more stories for children to practise with Anna Assertive.

Anna Assertive

29 Listening skills

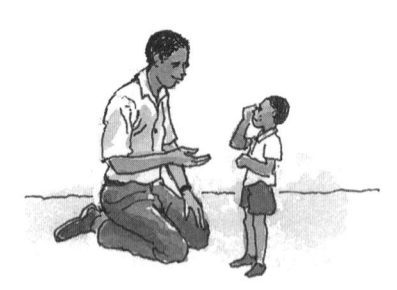

The importance of listening

Just as it is important to learn to be assertive and to speak clearly and calmly about what is important to us, so it is important to learn to listen.

As we have seen in Topic 17 (pages 36–37), being listened to can help young people to make healthy decisions and to stay safe from HIV and AIDS. Listening to another person shows respect. People who do not listen often want to dominate another person and feel that that person is not worth listening to. It is important that we teach children about listening and that we are role models of good listeners ourselves.

A good listener

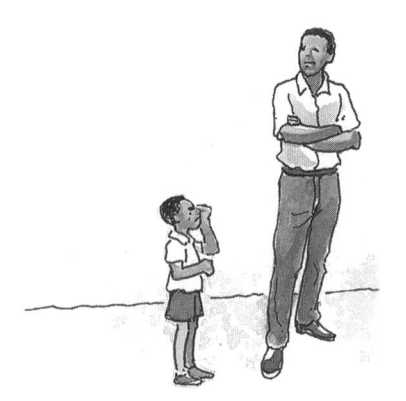

A bad listener

Helpful hints

At the beginning of the year, discuss with your class the importance of listening. Ask them to think about a time when they felt that someone did not listen to them. How did it feel? Ask them to think about a time when they did feel listened to. How did that feel?

Now let them complete this list.
A good listener:

- never interrupts
- waits for the other person to finish speaking before they respond
- wants to hear what the other person is saying
- shows that they are interested and that they care.

Now ask the class to make some rules for good listening for the rest of the year. Write them out and put them up in the classroom.

Activity Something to discuss

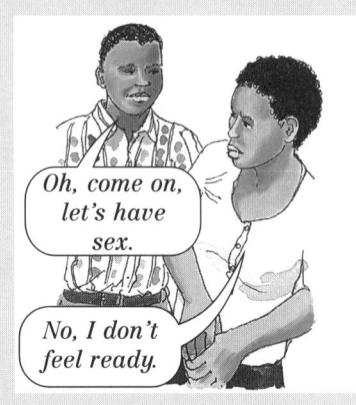

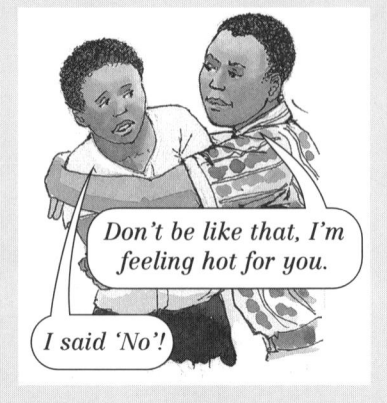

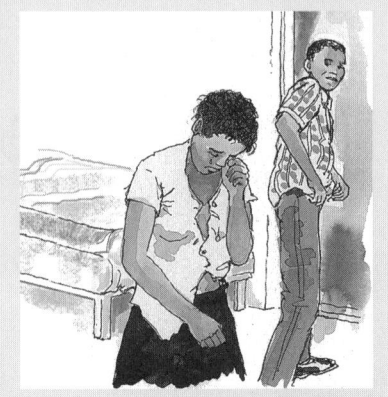

Oh, come on, let's have sex.

No, I don't feel ready.

Don't be like that, I'm feeling hot for you.

I said 'No'!

- What happened here?
- Why do you think the boy did not take the girl's 'No!' seriously?
- Do you think this happens often? Why?
- Sometimes boys think that when a girl says 'no' she means 'yes'. Why? How can you help change this?
- Males are often worse listeners than females. Why do you think this is so?
- How can we help the boys in our class to become better listeners?
- Do you think that people in your community listen to children enough?

Preventing the spread of HIV and AIDS

Ideas for the classroom

Here is a game to help children become aware of how difficult it can be to hear properly and to introduce the topic of listening.

1 Ask four of your better pupils to go outside, to be messengers.
2 Read a message to the children in the classroom once only. Ask one of the messengers outside to come in again.
3 Let a child volunteer to pass on the message to the messenger.
4 The next messenger comes in and the first messenger passes on the message.
5 Do this until the fourth messenger has repeated the message back to the whole group.
6 Read the original message again.
7 Discuss with the class what happened to the message. Did it get changed? If it did, why?
8 Talk to the children about how it is sometimes difficult to listen and to remember the facts. Also, talk about how important it is to listen carefully when we hear about AIDS and to make sure that we do not change the facts.

> **The message**
> Please ask Anna to tell Peter that he must bring his ruler to school tomorrow. If Anna does not see Peter, she must tell John to tell Peter about it. If she sees John, please tell him also to bring scissors.

Wrong information can kill!

Now show the pictures of the boy who did not listen to his girlfriend to the class. Use it to help teach them about being good listeners.

1 Divide the group into groups of boys and girls.
2 Boys should answer these questions.
   a Why do you think the boy did not listen to the girl?
   b What is it like when someone does not listen to you properly?
   c What is it like when someone listens to you?
   d Why do you think boys sometimes don't listen properly to girls?
   e How can we help boys to become better listeners?

Encourage them to think about the idea that listening is a way to show respect and how, when we don't listen, we sometimes want to prove that we are better than another person. Link this to the discussion about having good relationships.

3 Girls should answer these questions.
   a Why do you think the boy did not listen to the girl?
   b What is it like when someone does not listen to you properly?
   c What is it like when someone listens to you?
   d Why do you think boys sometimes don't listen properly to girls?
   e How can we make sure that boys hear girls?

Encourage the group to think about how listening is a way to show respect. How can girls be more assertive and make sure that they are heard? Link this to a discussion about having good relationships.

30 Resisting peer pressure

Definition

Peer pressure is pressure that children feel to behave in the same way they think their friends and other people their age (their peers) are behaving.

Young people and peer pressure

Even when we are adult, we experience pressure from our friends and peers to do things we don't really want to.

It is usually very hard to stand up against peer pressure because we like to be recognised and liked. We want to feel that we belong somewhere. We are afraid of being mocked and left out.

As young people begin to separate themselves from their parents, these feelings are especially strong. Young people also often form groups of friends. These groups can put a lot of pressure on them to act in certain ways.

What? You have never had sex! We've all had sex with many girls already.

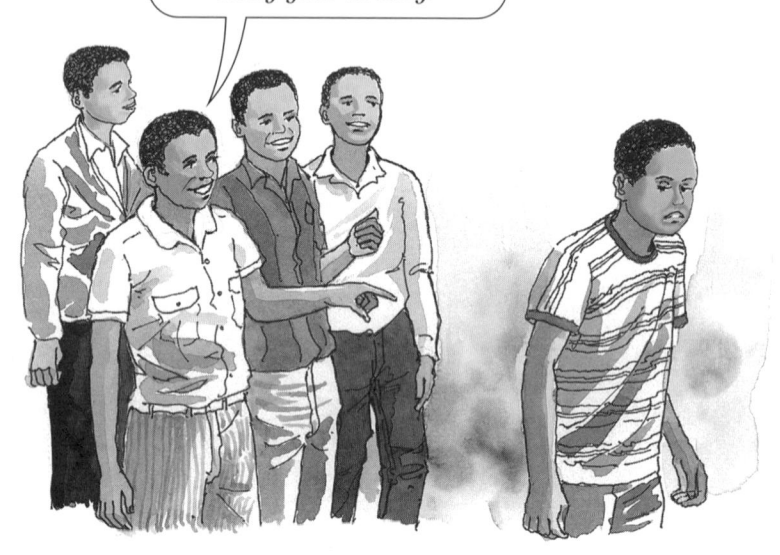

Activity Remembering your own experiences

To help you to teach about peer pressure, it is useful to remember how strong this type of pressure is. Try to remember your own youth.

- When you were young, did you belong to a group?
- What types of things did you do together?
- How did belonging to that group make you feel?
- Do you remember ever putting pressure on your peers to do things they did not want to do?

Helping children resist peer pressure

To help children deal with peer pressure, adults need to:

- help them to understand peer pressure and how it works
- help children build assertiveness skills and self-esteem
- encourage them to have healthy friendships
- encourage them to join youth clubs.

Think about when last you did something because you felt pressure from a friend. How did you feel? What made it hard to resist the pressure? Did you worry about what that person would think of you? Did you want to please that person?

Preventing the spread of HIV and AIDS

Anna Assertive is a puppet, made out of an old sock. See Topic 28, pages 60–61.

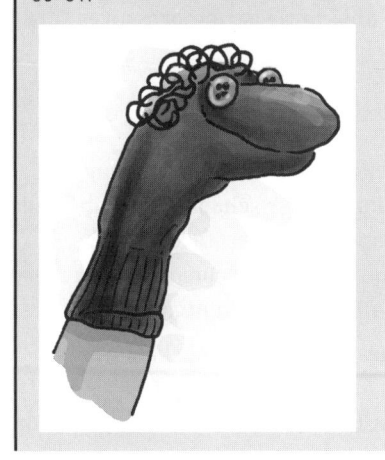

Ideas for the classroom

How to deal with peer pressure

Ask the children if they belong to a group of friends. How does that make them feel? What would happen if they did not want to do something that the group wants to do?

Explain peer pressure to the children and then let them do the following exercise. It involves three situations that Anna Assertive finds herself in. Let the children role-play them and suggest how she should respond.

1. Anna Assertive is shopping with her friends. It is very hot and they don't have money. One friend suggests they steal an ice cream.
2. Anna Assertive's best friend wants to go to a bar to meet a boy. Her parents will not allow her to go on her own. She asks Anna Assertive to lie for her and to say that Anna is going along.
3. Anna Assertive has an older brother. His friends are visiting for the weekend. Anna Assertive really likes to be with them. Anna Assertive goes with the boys to a dance. They buy her a beer.

Let the children work in groups and discuss which of the options in the box (left) would be the best thing to do in each case described.

Play the 'I say' game

Children stand in a circle. The teacher makes a statement that is typical of peer pressure. The statement starts with: 'I say.' The teacher throws a ball and the child who catches the ball responds for Anna Assertive. Here are some examples.

Teacher: I say: 'Let's go and steal some fruit.'
Anna Assertive: No thanks. I don't want to come along.

Teacher: I say: 'Let's drink some beer.'
Anna Assertive: No thanks, I prefer a soft drink.

Teacher: I say: 'If you really love me you will do what I say.'
Anna Assertive: If you love me, you will respect my answer.

Teacher: I say: 'You are just scared of your mother.'
Anna Assertive: I respect my mother and she trusts me to know how to behave.

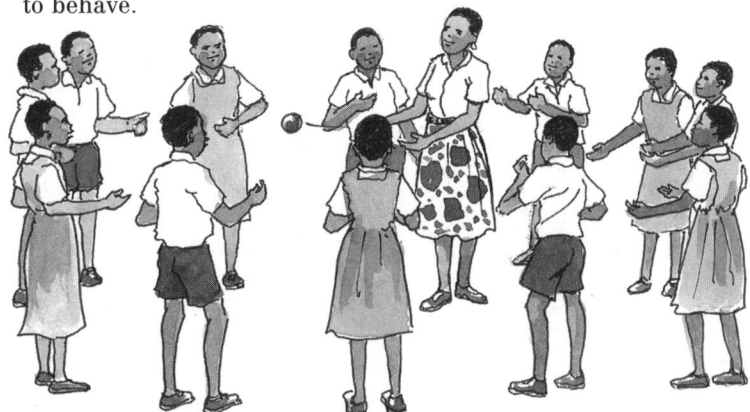

What could Anna do?

How could Anna respond to the situations described on this page?

Anna Assertive could **refuse**:
- No, I really don't want to.
- No, I am leaving now.
- No, I am not doing that.

Anna Assertive could **delay**:
- I am not ready now – maybe later.
- Maybe we can talk later.
- I'd like to talk to a friend first.

Anna Assertive could **bargain**:
- Lets do ...... instead.
- How about we try ......
- What would make us both happy?

31 Starting a Youth HIV and AIDS club

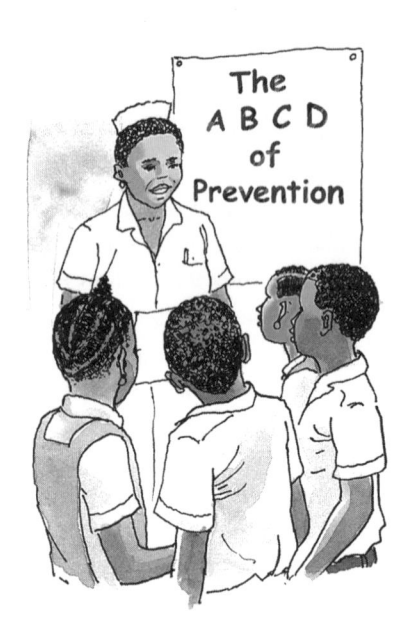

Changing the way young people behave is difficult. It takes time to help them to be more assertive and able to resist the pressures they face to have sex.

What a club can do

A very effective way to help them to stay healthy is by promoting the formation of a Youth HIV and AIDS club at your school. This club would promote healthy and safe behaviour and give accurate knowledge about health issues, especially HIV and AIDS. They could also form an abstinence club. The Youth HIV and AIDS club could organise:

- activities to encourage assertiveness and other life skills
- visits to health centres
- talks by professional people about HIV and AIDS and other health issues including STDs
- talks by people who are living with HIV and AIDS
- school health days
- support for those who are living with HIV and AIDS
- a vegetable-growing project to help those who need extra food.

Ideas for the classroom

In the lower primary classes, you could introduce the idea of HIV and AIDS activism by letting children prepare a campaign to promote the ABCD message to the rest of the school. Divide the class into groups and let each group deal with one aspect of the topic. To do this they could draw posters, which they can display at the school. They could also perform short dramas at assembly.

Let the pupils prepare a few clear messages about their topic for assembly. Here are some suggestions.

- **Abstain**

Delaying sex is safe and healthy. Your body does not need sex to grow. Sex is not safe for primary school children. If you have started sex already, you can start delaying again. Sex can make girls pregnant. Sex is not the same as love.

- **Be faithful**

Not having sex is your safest choice. If you have started sex, or when you are older, you need to speak to your partner openly about faithfulness and preventing pregnancy. You and your partner need to test for HIV. If you are both uninfected, you will be safe – as long as you only have sex with each other. If one or both of you are infected, you should talk to a health worker or counsellor about what you should do.

- **Condomise**

When you are older and get a partner, you need to talk about how to stay safe and test for HIV before you have sex. Condoms can reduce your risk of getting HIV and can prevent pregnancy.

Remember

Research shows that, when young people actively help those with HIV and AIDS, they are more likely to follow precautions and advice.

Preventing the spread of HIV and AIDS

- **Disease**

Stay free from sexually transmitted diseases (STDs) by abstaining, being faithful and by using condoms. If you do get a disease, get it treated quickly. Ask yourself: Is what I am doing good for my health? (See also Topic 39, pages 84–85).

Older children could discuss how to form a youth HIV and AIDS club at their school, and could get ideas from youth clubs in their area.

As a teacher, it is important that you help guide this process. Make sure that there are boys and girls in the club. Some people might have a bad attitude towards this club, so you, another teacher, or a responsible adult should attend all meetings, just as there is usually a responsible adult present at other types of youth clubs. Some people may even think that girls who join youth clubs are 'loose'.

Talk about these issues with the club members and help them to solve problems. As teacher, your role should be:

- guiding, encouraging and giving ideas to make sure that the club works. Help with sorting out any problems.
- distributing literature, which young people can read to improve their Life Skills and their knowledge about HIV and AIDS.
- helping link the club up with experts, other clubs and organisations which deal with HIV and AIDS and Life Skills.
- helping them draw up a practical action plan that will make sure that something is achieved.

How to form a Youth HIV/AIDS Club

1. Interested members meet and decide on the purpose of the Club.
2. They choose a chairperson and a secretary.
3. They can also choose a teacher who would help them when it is necessary.
4. They think of creative ways to encourage others to join.
5. They draw up an action plan for the next six months.

Here is an example:

The Good Shepherd Youth HIV and AIDS Club Action plan for first half year		
Date	Action	Who is responsible
26 January	Planning meeting	Everyone
3 April	AIDS Awareness march	The organising committee: Kofi, Susan, Patience, Hope
20 May	Meet with other Youth AIDS Clubs	Susan, Hope, Musa, Mandy
1 June	Organise talk by clinic sister on HIV prevention	John, Amina, Hope

Peer educators

In many countries it has been found that it is very useful to train young people themselves to spread the message of preventing the spread of HIV and AIDS. Young people are much more relaxed when they listen to other young people. These young peer educators are under careful supervision of teachers and counsellors.

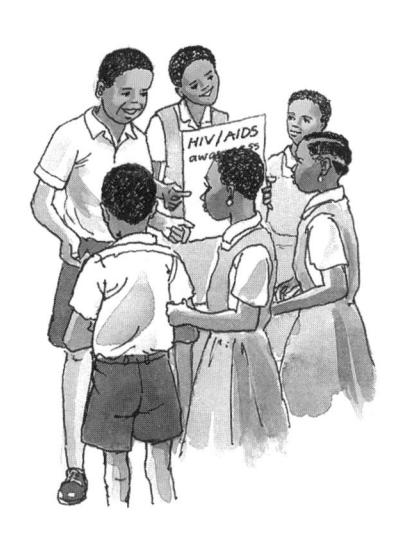

Section 4 Sex and sexuality

32 Our attitudes to sexuality

Definitions

Sex is the word used when we say whether we are male or female. The word is also used to describe two people having **sexual intercourse**.

Sexuality is the word used to speak about how we feel about sex and how we behave sexually. It is used when we discuss our attitudes to sex. Sexuality has different parts: sexual identity; reproduction and sexual health; sensuality; and intimacy.

Sexual identity is a term used when we want to talk about how we see ourselves, sexually. This includes how we feel about being a male or a female and what we think it means to be a man or a woman. It is also about what we have learnt from our community about being male and female.

Reproduction and **sexual health** are words used when we discuss our attitudes and behaviour about producing children. They are also used when we talk about looking after our body and our private parts and making sure that we do not catch sexually transmitted diseases (STDs).

Sensuality a word used to describe how we feel about our bodies. It is about whether we feel attractive and sexy. It is about whether we enjoy using our bodies, for example by doing sport. Do we like to dress in a way attractive to others? Do we find other people attractive?

Intimacy is being able to be emotionally close to another person. It is about enjoying sharing with another person and liking them. It can also be between friends or between parents and children, and so may not have anything to do with sex at all.

What do you feel when you hear the word 'sex'? Curious? Afraid? Excited? Confused? Happy? Angry? Disappointed? Sad? Lonely?

This is a topic which has confused and delighted people for a long time – perhaps always! People usually have different, and often mixed-up, feelings about it.

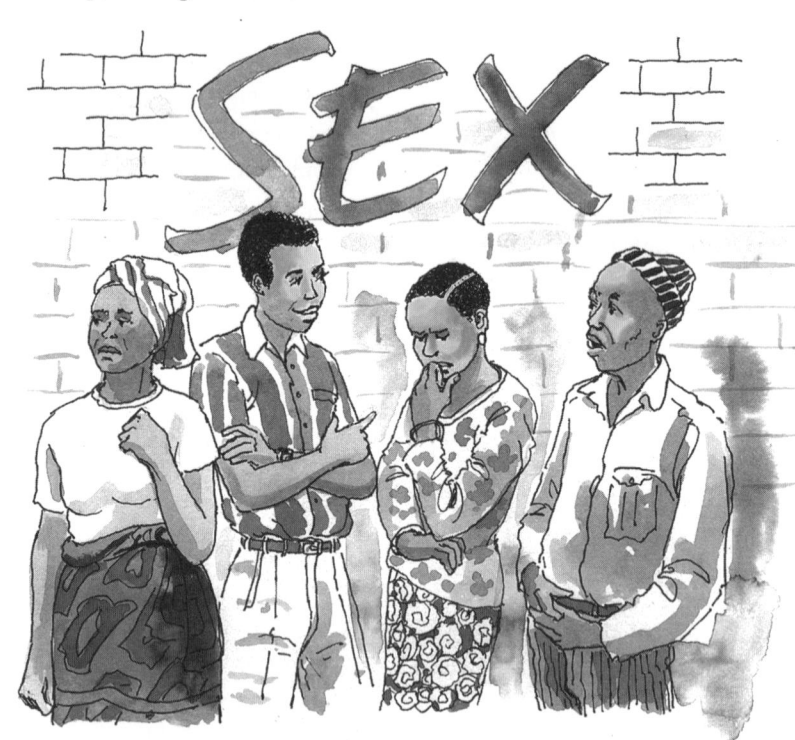

What do you feel about the word 'sex'.

Ideas for the classroom

Encourage your pupils to think about attitudes to men and women in their community. This could be related to work in Social Studies. Talk with them about proverbs or 'sayings' relating to men and women. What qualities are seen as good in men and women?

Boys can investigate how boys are taught to be men. Girls can investigate how girls are taught to be women.

Groups of boys and girls can present their findings to the whole class.

Discuss adults' attitudes to the ways girls and boys behave. Have the children noticed any differences?

Sex and sexuality

The importance of sexuality

Sexuality is a natural and important part of who we are, from when we are born until we die. It can be used positively to attract a partner or negatively to control or harm another person. Most cultures and communities have made many rules about it. Often these rules are about not speaking about sex. Some of these rules are useful, but others can cause confusion and harm people.

Helpful hint

Children are generally even more confused and embarrassed about sexuality than we adults are. To help them to develop a healthy sexuality, it is important that you learn to be relaxed and clear when you speak about issues such as sex and sexuality. It helps to stick to accurate and clear facts. Be well informed. Keep the conversations friendly and natural.

Activity Thinking about our attitudes to sex and sexuality

Here are some questions to help you think about your community's attitude to sexuality and how it affects your teaching about HIV and AIDS. You may want to discuss these questions with your colleagues at school.

Sensuality
How are boys in your society encouraged to show that they enjoy their bodies? How are girls encouraged to show that they enjoy their bodies? Are girls allowed to show their sensuality as much as boys are? Are married women allowed to show their sensuality in the same way as unmarried women? And married men? What are the rules of flirtation in your society? Are girls encouraged to flirt with boys?

Intimacy
How is emotional intimacy encouraged between husband and wife? Are they encouraged to have a friendship, or is the husband supposed to have all the power? Are things changing in your community?

Sexual identity
How are boys taught to be men in your community? How are girls taught to be women? Who teaches them? Is there formal teaching (e.g. initiation schools)? Or is it done informally by parents and peers? Has this changed since you were young? What is your society's attitude to homosexuality?

Sexual health and reproduction
How did you learn about reproduction? How are boys and girls today taught about reproduction? How were girls in the past taught about menstruation?

Your own society
What are the most positive aspects of your society's attitudes to sexuality? What are the most negative aspects of your society's attitudes to sexuality? How do you think these attitudes would affect your teaching about HIV and AIDS?

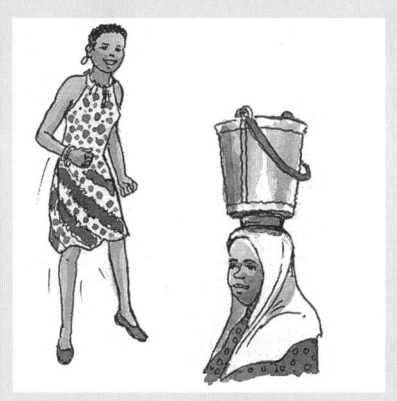

How does your society see the role of women?

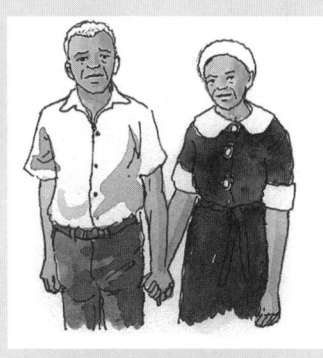

How do husbands and wives show intimacy?

33 Teaching about sex

Remember!

Sex education does **not** encourage children to have sex. It can help them to make better decisions about sex and sexuality. When they are tempted or under pressure to have sex, it is not enough if they say: 'I am not allowed to have sex.' They need to be able to say: 'I choose for myself not to have sex.'

The different parts of sex education

Sex education has many parts. It is about teaching the biology of reproduction and about Life Skills such as communication and decision-making. It is about encouraging healthy and respectful relationships between men and women. It is also about the spiritual aspects of sex. It helps children to be assertive and feel good about their bodies.

Activity   Remember your own experience

Think about your own first sexual experience. Did you feel that you were ready? Did you have enough knowledge? What were the circumstances? Were you married to the person? What was confusing? What would you have liked to have known beforehand?

What stories about sex and reproduction were you told when you were young? What did adults tell you about where babies came from? Find out about local myths about how babies are made. For example, in some societies, parents tell children that babies are brought to them by a bird called a stork.

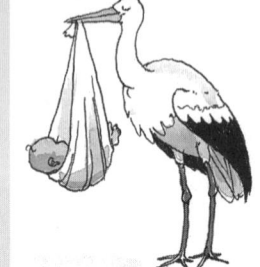

Think about your own sex education.

- Where did you get your information from?
- Was the information correct?
- What attitudes did it give you?
- How did it help you?
- How did it make things more difficult?
- How would you have liked to have learnt about sex and sexuality?

Now think about how you would teach a lesson about sexual intercourse.

Ideas for the classroom

Before teaching about human sexuality, it is useful to let children look at how everything in nature reproduces. Children need to feel and understand that sex is a very important and joyful part of nature. They can draw the life cycle of plants, animals, insects and people and then compare them.

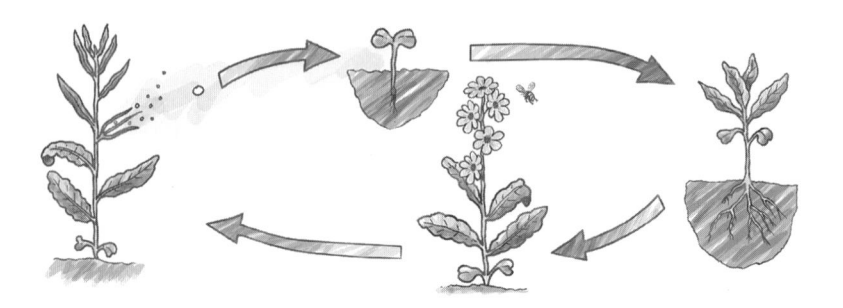

The life cycle of a plant

Sex and sexuality

Let the children talk or write about their experience of an animal (maybe a dog, cat or a cow) that had young.

They can talk or write about how they experienced the birth of a younger brother or sister. What happened to their mother? How did they feel?

Activity

Plan a series of lessons about reproduction for upper primary children. Think about how you will find out what the children know already. Think about the language you are going to use and teach. Think about the progression from one lesson to the next. How will you involve the children in learning rather than simply talking to them and explaining the facts?

Language

What language should we use to speak about HIV and AIDS?

In many cultures it is not acceptable to speak about sex and HIV and AIDS in the local language. Some teachers feel that they can use English words instead. However, because it is important to teach about HIV and AIDS from the early grades, there is a danger that young children may not understand English. It is important that your whole school decides on what to do about this. All teachers should agree and act in the same way so that no one teacher is seen as 'bad' or corrupting the children.

The next step would be to introduce children to the vocabulary of reproduction. Use factual and correct language so that you don't confuse the children. They need to be able to name all the body parts that are involved in reproduction and sexual organs. (See Topic 35, pages 74–75.)

The most important part is to actually teach the facts about human reproduction. This includes how people have sex, how babies are born and facts about menstruation and ejaculation. It is very important that you, as the teacher, are well informed about the facts of sexual intercourse and sexuality so that you do not pass on wrong information. (For a sample lesson on sexual intercourse look at Topic 38, pages 80–83.)

Helpful hints

- Use opportunities to speak to young children about sexuality when they ask questions related to sex and then take your time to explain. You can also speak about it after there has been a religious or cultural event such as a wedding, birth, baptism or a funeral.
- Some schools in Uganda have introduced a Health Letter Box. It is a box at the school where primary school children can put questions about sex they are too embarrassed to ask, without giving their names. For example they can ask questions about erections, wet dreams or about courtship. These questions are answered in assembly by trained teachers.
- Some schools also have teachers who can give counselling. For example, a male teacher could stay behind once a week to answer the boys' questions about reproductive health and relationships. A female teacher could do the same to help girls.

34 Teaching about sex at the right level

The problems of teaching young children

Sex education has to start from a very early age. What makes this difficult in the classroom is that some children may know a lot while others know very little. In some classes there are also older and younger children together.

Before you teach about sex and sexuality, it is important to listen to the children and to find out what they know already. You can also do a quick quiz to check their knowledge. Make sure that you answer any of the children's questions clearly and accurately. If you don't know the answer, find out and tell the children the answer later.

Try to find out how much the children in your class know about sex by listening carefully to how they themselves answer questions and the questions they ask.

It is important that your whole school discusses the issue of speaking about sex and HIV and AIDS with the children. This is so that teachers are united. The school needs to have a policy about this. Share this policy with the parents, and let them give their input. When drawing up this policy the school can think about these questions.

- What language do we use to talk about sex and sexuality? (See Topic 33, page 71.)
- What can we talk about at what age?
- How can we answer the questions our children have truthfully?
- Should we have an anonymous box where children can put questions? (See Topic 5, page 13 and Topic 33, page 71.)
- Who could we ask to help us with sexuality and HIV and AIDS education?

What can we talk about at what age?

People change physically and mentally throughout their lives. Here are some ideas about what you can discuss at what age. But also remember that each child is unique.

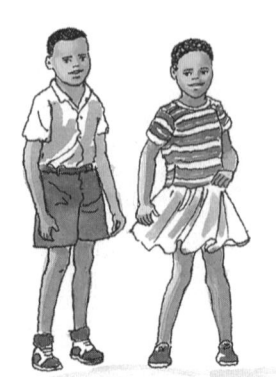

Children up to 9 years old

Young children are very curious. They will ask many questions. They need simple and accurate answers.

Give simple lessons about reproduction, linking it to the natural world. Young children need to know the names of all their body parts, including the penis and the vagina and what they are used for. Speak about keeping private parts clean and not letting anybody, except those who are close to them, touch them. Remind the children about good touching and bad touching (see Topic 21, pages 44–45).

Sex and sexuality

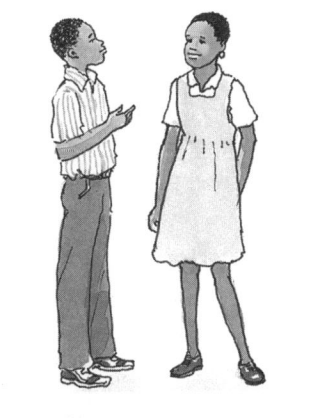

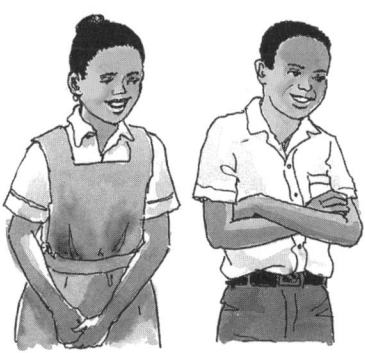

Children from 9 to 14 years

This is the beginning of puberty. It is a difficult time, and children need adults to be patient and understanding. Boys and girls need to understand the physical and emotional changes that are happening to them. Some start to be sexually active, and they need to know the facts about sexual intercourse and about the dangers of getting infected with HIV. (See Topic 35, pages 74–75, and Topic 39, pages 84–85.)

Girls, especially, need information so that they can stay safe from the sexual advances of older boys or men. This is because they develop earlier than boys and are often more vulnerable, because they may have been taught to be submissive to men. ((See Topic 7, page 17, Topic 28, pages 60–61, on assertiveness, etc. and Topic 40, pages 86–87.)

Children from 15 years and above

Many teenagers are sexually active. They may also not want to listen to adults. This makes them very vulnerable to falling pregnant and getting infected with HIV or other sexually transmitted diseases. At this stage they need to know as much as possible about reproduction, sexual health and healthy sexual behaviour. Teenagers want to be taken seriously and to be given responsibility. They benefit from peer sexuality education and from joining youth clubs. They also need to know where to get medical help and information. They need strong relationships with caring adults.

Helpful hints

- It is very important that you use correct and understandable words and information about sex. Incorrect information can confuse children and can put them at risk.
- It is also important to provide an opportunity for young people to ask questions without fear of ridicule. Here an anonymous question box is very useful. (See Topic 5, page 13 and Topic 33, page 71).

To deal with a variety of knowledge and experience around sex, it is useful to use group-work and peer education.

For example:

- You can group children according to age and experience.
- You can teach boys and girls separately. If possible, you and a colleague can share the teaching. Move all the girls into one class and the boys into another. You could also divide boys and girls into same-sex groups in one class.

Activity

With your colleagues share your experience of the kinds of questions your own children or your pupils have asked about sex.

How did you respond? Could you have responded better? Can you remember what questions you had about sex:

- Before you were 9?
- Between 9 and 14?
- Older than 15?

35 Puberty: the changing body

Definition
Most boys will occasionally have a sexy dream and ejaculate in the night while they are sleeping. This is called a **wet dream**. Boys can find this embarrassing, and need to know that it is natural and normal. It is the way that the body makes space for new sperm from the testicles. It does **not** mean that a boy must have sex.

Puberty

During puberty, the bodies of boys and girls change a lot. This can cause confusion. It is made worse because young people often compare themselves to others and worry that they are not normal.

It is important that you explain the changes in great detail, and that you reassure children that each one of us develops in our own time and at our own pace.

Boys and girls need to know about what happens to both sexes so that they can develop understanding and respect for each other. Boys need to know about menstruation and girls need to know about erections and wet dreams.

Boys

Most boys start to grow fast between the ages of 12 and 14. Usually it starts with the feet growing bigger, their shoulders grow wider and their legs longer. At this time the body produces a lot of testosterone. This is the male sex hormone that changes the body from a boy to a man.

- His muscles grow and he becomes stronger.
- He will start to develop body hair around the private parts, under the arms and on the chest.
- His voice becomes deeper.
- His penis and scrotum grow bigger.
- He will sweat more and the body smell will change.
- His skin may become oily and he can develop pimples.
- He gets more erections and he will start to release semen or ejaculate. (This means that if he has sexual intercourse with a girl he can make her pregnant.)

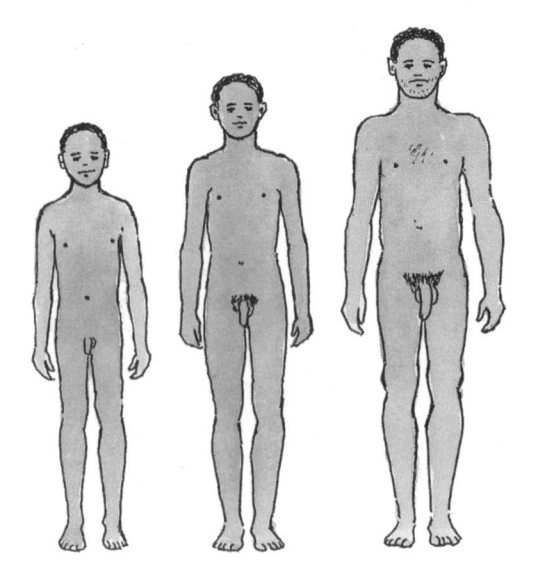

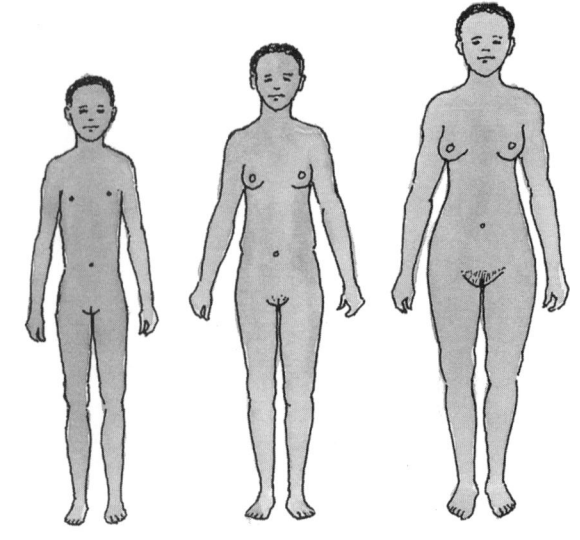

How boys develop (see also page 133)   *How girls develop (see also page 133)*

Sex and sexuality

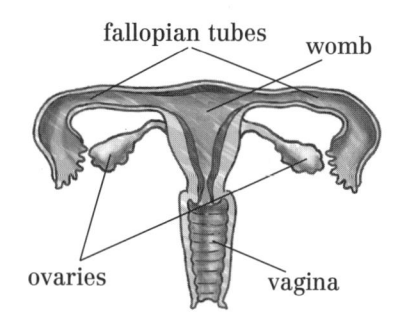

The female reproductive system (labels: fallopian tubes, womb, ovaries, vagina)

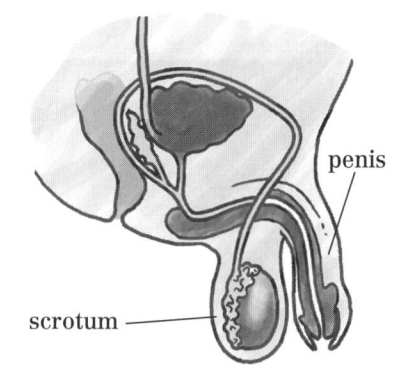

Male sex organs (labels: penis, scrotum)

Girls

Females usually begin to change from girls to women around the ages of 10 or 12. They reach puberty earlier than boys, which is why they need to be especially protected from the advances of older boys and men. Their bodies produce the female sex hormone, called oestrogen and begin to change.

- A girl develops breasts.
- Her hips get bigger.
- Hair starts to grow around her private parts and under her arms.
- She will sweat more and the body smells get stronger.
- Her skin gets oily and she can develop pimples.
- She will start to menstruate.

Menstruation

Most girls begin to menstruate between the ages of 10 and 16. Once this happens, a girl can become pregnant if she has sex with a male. It is possible for girls to become pregnant *before* the first period. Each month the ovaries each produce an egg. As the egg matures, it travels down the fallopian tubes to the uterus or womb. The uterus makes a thick lining so that the egg can grow. If the egg is not fertilised by a male's sperm, the lining is not needed and it breaks down and comes out of the vagina as blood. This bleeding is called **menstruation**. It is possible to get HIV before, after and during menstruation.

Ideas for the classroom

A good way to start teaching about the development of the sex organs during puberty is to divide the class into groups of boys and groups of girls. Let each group draw a picture of what they think a girl's and a boy's reproductive organs look like. Let them label them.

Either you or a teacher who specialises in biology or general science can look at the pictures. Then put up the correct drawings up and teach the functions and name of the organs. Now teach about the physical changes that happen during puberty.

Topic 36, pages 76–77 will help you to teach about the emotional changes that happen during puberty.

Helpful hint

To help children become more comfortable with talking openly about sexuality, write the following list of words on the board after the first sex education lesson.

scared	interested	tired	excited	negative	want to be alone
ashamed	not interested	happy	angry	confused	don't know
dirty	confident	worried	lonely	relieved	
nervous	disappointed	hot	in love	sad	
bored	disgusted	hurt	cheeky	shocked	
cold	jealous	embarrassed	sad	surprised	

Ask the children to choose the words that describe their feelings. They can also add their own words. Discuss the feelings with the class and explain that none of these feelings are bad.

36 Puberty: the changing personality

Becoming an adult

Puberty is the time when children begin to change into adults. As our bodies change, so do our feelings and the way that we relate to one another. It is useful for a teacher to understand these changes, so that you can understand and teach the children in your class about them.

Emotional changes

The same hormones that help to change the body from child to adult also affect the emotions. They can cause a lot of confusion. One moment the young person can feel very happy, but the next they can feel very depressed. A few days before they menstruate, girls often feel like crying or they are very depressed. Often, young people will withdraw from adults and keep secrets.

As girls and boys grow into puberty, they will have more sexual feelings. Boys will start having sexy dreams and wake up to find that they have ejaculated. They will discuss sex and girls with one another and may often brag about their sexual abilities. Girls may spend a lot of time talking about love, sex and boys to their friends.

Mental changes

At this time, young people generally want to start thinking for themselves and make their own decisions. They often ask critical questions about their culture and the way adults do things.

Relationship changes

For younger children, the home and family are very important. They need to feel that they belong. As they get into puberty, children pay less attention to adults – their friends and peers become more important. This can cause fighting and unhappiness in the home. Children can become rebellious.

Younger children also are not so aware of the difference between boys and girls, but as they get older they may not want to play with each other any more and they may become shy and embarrassed. Later, this changes again.

Worry about appearance

During puberty, children are often very embarrassed about the changes that are happening to their bodies. They will compare themselves to others and worry about whether they are normal. Some children will spend a lot of time in front of the mirror and be very critical of what they see, and feel ugly. This happens especially to girls, who wonder whether they are pretty enough. Boys can often worry about whether their penises are large enough.

Sex and sexuality

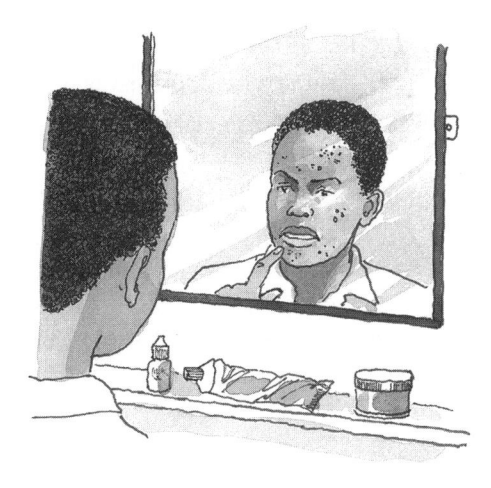

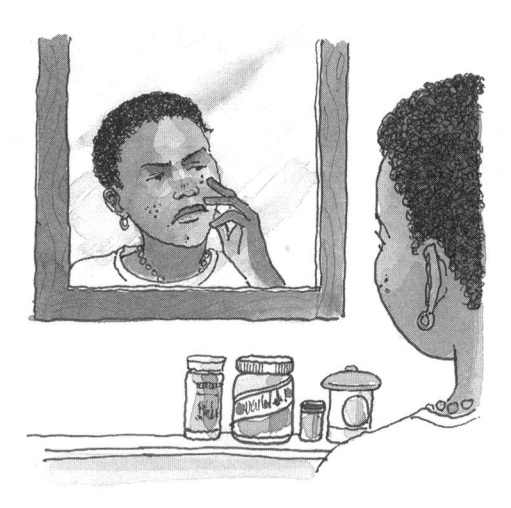

Activity Thinking about puberty among your pupils

To be able to help the children in your class on a more individual level, think about which of the changes outlined on the opposite page you recognise in them. (See Topic 35, pages 74–75.) Are there any ways in which you could reassure and support them in the classroom?

It is important to reassure children. Girls need to be given confidence. They need to hear the message that their body is theirs and that being a woman is something to be proud of.

Boys also need to be given confidence and reassurance that everyone develops differently and that each penis looks different.

Ideas for the classroom

Show the children pictures on page 74 of boys and girls at different stages of development. If the children have access to newspapers or magazines they could cut out their own pictures of young people. Allow the children to talk in groups about what is happening to the people in the picture, physically and emotionally.

They can revise what they learnt about physical changes and begin to discuss emotional changes. You can guide them by asking questions such as: 'What do you think each person in the picture worries about most in their life?' 'What do you think their relationship is with their parents?' 'What do you think they feel about people of the other sex?'

Now go through the changes discussed above and link them to how they can make a person vulnerable to getting infected with HIV and AIDS. For example, physical changes can make the children have sexual feelings. It is dangerous just to act on these feelings. Link this discussion with abstinence. (See Topic 25, pages 52–53.)

Because of the confusion that is caused by emotional and physical changes it is important to encourage positive goal setting and improving self-esteem. (See Topic 23, page 48.)

Some of these changes can make children more vulnerable to peer pressure and to unprotected sex. (See Topic 30, pages 64–65.)

Helpful hint

Adults are often not prepared for the changes that children go through, and may get angry when children no longer listen to them. They may want to force them to obey. But this is the time when children really need guidance from adults – not judgement or conflict.

37 Dealing with sexual feelings

Feeling sexy (having sexual feelings) is something that most people experience from time to time. Sexual feelings are those we get when we find another person attractive.

Arousal

Often these feelings cause arousal. When a boy is aroused his penis will be erect. When a girl is aroused her vagina will get wet. Sexual feelings can come from thinking about a person we find attractive, from looking at sexy pictures or movies and from reading a love story. We can also be aroused by touching and hugging someone we find attractive.

Ideas for the classroom

It is important that all children learn that being sexually aroused does not mean that they must have sex. To stay safe children need to know about abstinence (see Topic 25, pages 52–53) and self-control.

Older children should be taught to decide beforehand how far they will go if they are in a situation where there could be sex. This is because sexual activity is often not planned and, sometimes, it is difficult to refuse.

Ask both boys and girls to think about these questions for when they are in a situation where there might be sex:

Will you let the other person

- Kiss you?
- Hug you?
- Hold hands?
- Touch your private parts/breasts?

What will you do if they do something you don't want?

Be clear that it is safest not to do these things. Tell children that it can be very difficult to stop once sexual feelings are aroused. Also, explain that if people have drunk alcohol it may be even more difficult. Encourage children to find other activities to keep them busy, such as sport, music, belonging to youth clubs or craft work.

Children, especially girls, can often confuse sexual feelings with being in love. In some cultures 'Proposing love' means offering to have sex. It is therefore important to help children to look at what it means when someone says 'I love you'.

Put the children into boys' and girls' groups. Ask them to write down as many ways as possible of saying that you are interested in someone from the opposite sex. For example, 'I fancy you.' 'I love you.' 'Will you be my girl?'

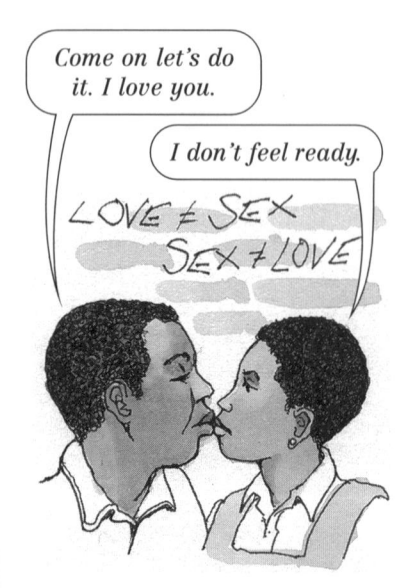

Sex and sexuality

Now ask them to talk about what these expressions mean in terms of what the other person wants. Do they want to get to know you better? Do they want to have sex? Do they want to be faithful to you? Are they showing you the type of love that goes with respect?

Let the groups report back. It is important to point out that when someone says 'I love you' it does not mean you must have sex with them. And if you say 'I love you' it does not mean you are willing to have sex. Children need to understand that having sex has to be agreed on properly by both people beforehand. People should not only be above the age of consent, but should really be adult, test for HIV, and agree to remain faithful, before they have sex.

Refer children to what they learnt about healthy relationships in Topic 26, pages 56–57, and how to show feelings without having sex in Topic 25, pages 52–53.

Important information for teachers – 1

Masturbation

This is another way to show sexual feelings.

It is important that you as a teacher know the facts about masturbation. This is when we touch our own sexual organs such as the penis, vagina, breasts or other parts of the body that are sensitive, to reach orgasm. Most people masturbate at some time during their lives. It does not harm the body.

Some people say it is better to masturbate than to risk pregnancy or getting HIV and AIDS, but some cultures give wrong information about masturbation.
Here are some examples:

- You can go mad if you masturbate. ✗
- It can make you grow hair on the palms of your hands. ✗
- It can make you weak and makes you lose interest in sex. ✗

If children do ask about masturbation, and you feel comfortable talking about it, they need to know that:

- Many cultures and religions do not approve of it.
- It is a safer way to show sexual feelings than having sex.
- It can help with abstinence.
- It is not physically harmful, unless it becomes an addiction – that is, if a person feels that they cannot go through the day without masturbating.

Activity

Reflect on your own attitudes to:

- masturbation
- homosexuality.

Do you think your attitudes are the same as your colleagues?

Important information for teachers – 2

Homosexuality

It is important that you, as a teacher, know about homosexuality. You do not need to teach about it if you are uncomfortable about it, or if it is against school policy to do so.

Some people feel attracted to people of the same sex. Men can be attracted to other men and women can be attracted to women. Many people have these feelings at some time of their life. Some people are attracted to people of their own sex throughout their lives. Many cultures and religions are against homosexuality and feel that a person with these feelings can be changed or ought to change. Others disagree and say that homosexuality is something a person is born with and that they cannot control or change.

38 Teaching about sexual intercourse and pregnancy

Keeping to the facts

When children ask questions about sex, remember that it is important to answer them correctly, and not to mix the facts with moralising about sex.

> ### Important information for teachers – 1
>
> **The facts about having sex**
>
> Sexual intercourse, or sex, is when a male puts his penis inside another person. Before intercourse, as the male gets more excited his penis gets hard and starts to produce lubricating liquid. The female's vagina, into which the male puts his penis, will also swell and produce liquids. These allow the penis to slide into the vagina more easily.
>
> After a while, there usually is an orgasm, or climax. When a male has an orgasm, his muscles contract and he pushes out a liquid called semen from his penis. This contains the sperm or seeds. A woman may also have an orgasm, and the muscles around her vagina may contract. If the sperm fertilises an egg, which is produced by the female's body, she will fall pregnant.

> ### Important information for teachers – 2
>
> **HIV and sex**
>
> If a person carries HIV, their sexual liquids can infect their partner.
>
> - The liquid that the penis produces before the male ejaculates contains some sperm, and so can cause pregnancy. HIV is carried in the semen, and can infect the female. Babies may get infected through the mother's blood if she has HIV or AIDS.
> - If a girl is afraid or forced to have sex she will not produce sexual liquid in her vagina. Some cultures use herbs to dry and tighten the woman's vagina during sex, so that the man can enjoy sex more. A dry vagina can be more easily damaged than a wet one, and this makes a woman more vulnerable to getting infected with HIV.
> - Oral sex is when people stimulate each other's private parts with the mouth or tongue. HIV can be passed on in this way if there are sores or cuts in the mouth.
> - Anal sex is when the penis is put inside the anus. HIV can be spread easily in this way, as the skin inside the anus can tear very easily.
> - Mutual masturbation is when two people give each other orgasm by using hands and fingers to stimulate each other. HIV is not passed on in this way unless there are open wounds on the hands.

Sex and sexuality

> *Remember*
> When teaching about sexual intercourse you will have to decide what is appropriate for the age of the children and for your community. But remember that keeping children safe is most important.

Ideas for the classroom

The introductory lesson that follows is suitable for Upper Primary School children, and should follow a discussion of sexual feelings and relationships.

Sample lesson about sex

Introduction

Talk about weddings. Why are they such important and happy events? Guide the conversation towards the idea that people often get married because they want to start a family.

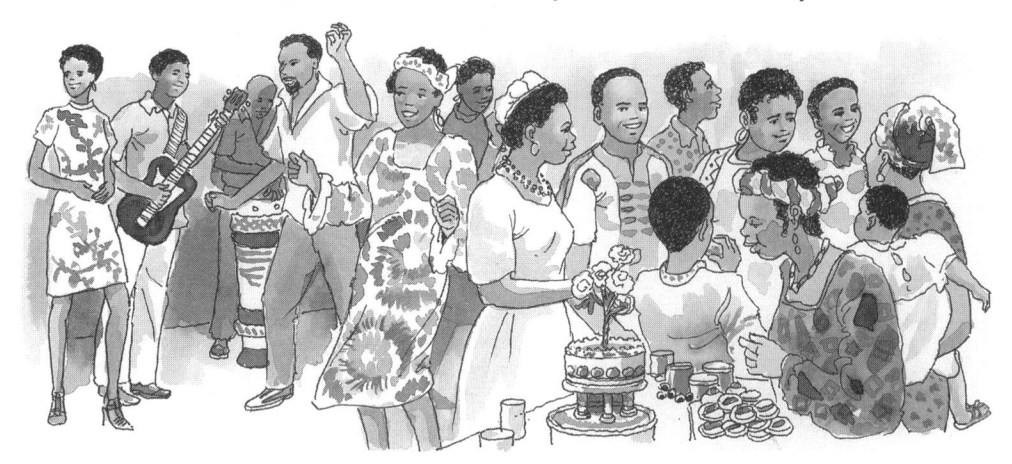

Main lesson

Lead on from the introduction with questions such as, 'How do people make children?' The answer is that people have sexual intercourse.

How does this happen?

1 A man and a woman get sexually excited. They touch each other and kiss. The man's penis gets hard. This is called an erection. The woman's vagina gets wet.
2 The man puts his penis into the vagina and moves it until he gets an orgasm. This is when his muscles pump semen into the vagina.
3 In the semen, there is the seed or sperm. This seed travels up the vagina. If it finds an egg that is ready, it will fertilise it and the woman will become pregnant.

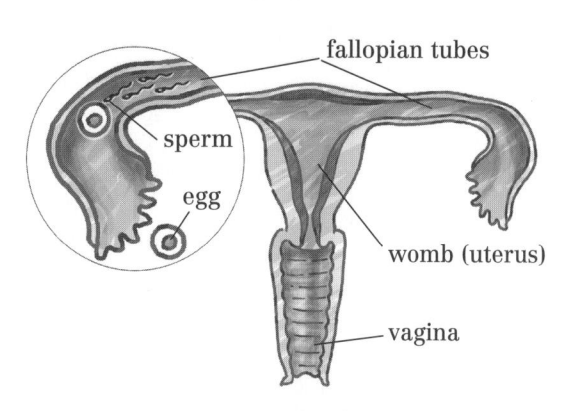

Teaching about HIV and AIDS

Make sure you answer any questions that the children have about this process, especially those that that will help them stay safe.

Conclusion

Link this lesson with HIV and AIDS. Make sure that children understand clearly the link between having sex and getting HIV and AIDS. Talk about using condoms, staying faithful and getting tested before having sex. Also, talk about the fact that there are other diseases that one can get from having sex. (See Topic 39, pages 84–85.)

> *Helpful hint*
>
> If you find out that a child knows too much about sexual intercourse for his or her age, it can be a sign that the child has been sexually abused. Get help. Don't try to solve this on your own.

Teaching about pregnancy

Children need to know that getting pregnant in primary school can be very dangerous. A young girl's body is often not developed enough, and can be damaged when the baby is born. Her vagina can tear badly, or it might have to be cut to allow the baby to come out. Young girls are more likely to die giving birth than older women.

In addition, the girl's education is interrupted, and she will also face the emotional and economic difficulties of having a child when she is too young to be able to cope with either.

It is very important that children of all ages understand that having sex can make a girl pregnant.

Try the quiz below. If you know of any wrong ideas that the children have, add them to this quiz. Answer 'True' or 'False'.

Discuss the answers afterwards. (You can find the correct answers on pages 130 and 131.)

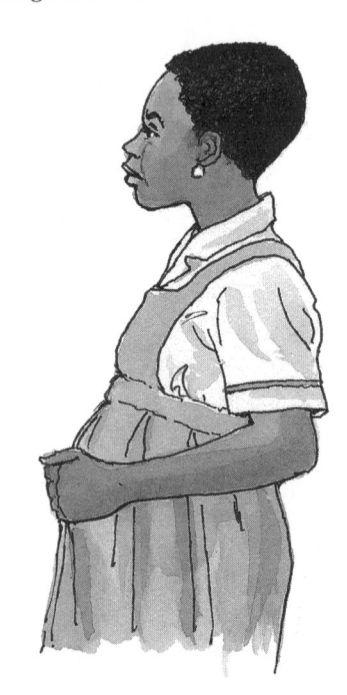

> *Quiz*
>
> 1 You can't get pregnant if you have sex standing up.
> 2 You will not get pregnant if the boy pulls out before he ejaculates.
> 3 You can't get pregnant if you have sex when you are menstruating.
> 4 You can't get pregnant if you wash yourself properly after sex.
> 5 A 12-year-old boy cannot make a girl pregnant.
> 6 Only bad girls get pregnant.
> 7 There is a pill that can stop a girl from getting pregnant and getting HIV.
> 8 You can't get pregnant from only having sex once.

Sex and sexuality

Helpful hints

It is very important that boys learn to **take responsibility for pregnancy**. It is useful if a male teacher discusses this with the boys separately. You need to get these points across:

- A boy is just as responsible as a girl for a pregnancy.
- There are no safe days on which to have sex with a girl.
- Pregnancy can be dangerous for your girlfriend.
- Pregnancy can spoil the chances of a boy and a girl getting a good education.
- If you do become a father you must take responsibility and help the girl.

Some facts about pregnancy

A woman can know that she is pregnant when she misses her menstrual period. This is because the lining of the womb stays inside and makes a nest for the baby to grow in. Sometimes she can miss her period without being pregnant. Other signs of pregnancy are:

- sore breasts
- feeling nauseous
- being tired all the time
- needing to urinate often.

The only certain way of knowing is to take a pregnancy test.

Pregnancy normally takes 40 weeks. The baby grows very fast in the beginning. When it is 12 weeks old it already looks like a human being with a very big head.

A pregnant woman needs to look after herself well. She should not drink or smoke. She needs healthy food and lots of rest.

Pregnancy and HIV

It is very important that a mother protects herself from HIV infection while she is pregnant. This is because, if she is infected, she can pass the infection on to her baby. About 30 per cent of babies whose mothers are infected are also infected with HIV.

There is medicine available that a woman who is infected with HIV can take. It reduces the chances of giving the infection to the baby.

It is also better not to breastfeed your baby, if you are infected with HIV, because there is a risk of transmitting HIV through breast milk.

It is important that children think about these questions. They should not answer them out loud, just think about them.

- Do you want to have children?
- How many children do you want to have?
- When do you want to have children?
- What do you need to do, to prepare for having children?

39 Teaching about HIV and AIDS and other STDs

> **Did you know?**
>
> Some sexually transmitted diseases (diseases spread through sexual contact) – like syphilis and gonorrhoea – are serious diseases, but they can usually be managed and cured. HIV and AIDS are the worst STD you can get, as these have no cure.

HIV and AIDS

Young people have always experimented with sex. The HIV and AIDS epidemic has made this natural and exciting part of growing up much more risky, because having sex can kill.

It is important that children understand that the main way that one can get HIV and AIDS is through having sex. HIV is a sexually transmitted disease (STD).

Other diseases

There are many other types of infections and diseases that are passed on through sex. These include gonorrhoea, chlamydia, syphilis, genital warts and genital herpes. What helps some STDs, and especially HIV, spread more easily is that many people who are infected do not show any symptoms at first. Young people need to know how to stay safe from STDs. (See Topics 24–27, pages 50–59.)

Some STDs do have symptoms and young people need to recognise them:

Signs in girls and women

These can include:

- discharge or fluid from the vagina that is thick, itchy or has a strong smell. It can be green or yellow. To recognise this girls need to know that normal discharge is clear or whitish. It smells healthy and is not itchy
- itching in the genital area
- pain in the lower abdomen or when urinating
- abnormal or irregular bleeding from the vagina
- pain during sexual intercourse
- swelling, sores or growths in the genital area.

Signs in boys and men

These can include:

- sores, rashes or blisters on and around the penis
- yellow discharge from the penis
- pain when urinating
- pain and swelling of the testicles and swellings or growths on the genitals.

The links between HIV and AIDS and other STDs

Sores and breaks in the skin caused by STDs can increase the risk of getting and passing on HIV and AIDS. In addition, having an STD shows that the person has had unprotected sex. This means that they are at risk of having HIV, although they may not know they have it.

> **Did you know?**
>
> Girls are more vulnerable than boys to getting STDs, including HIV and AIDS. This is because the sexual fluids of a man stay inside a girl's body longer. Also, the cervix and vagina of young girls can tear during sex, and this can be made more likely by cultural practices such as putting herbs or cloths inside the vagina to dry or tighten it. Women are also more at risk of having unwanted sex. It can also be difficult for them to protect themselves from STDs by insisting that a condom is used.

Sex and sexuality

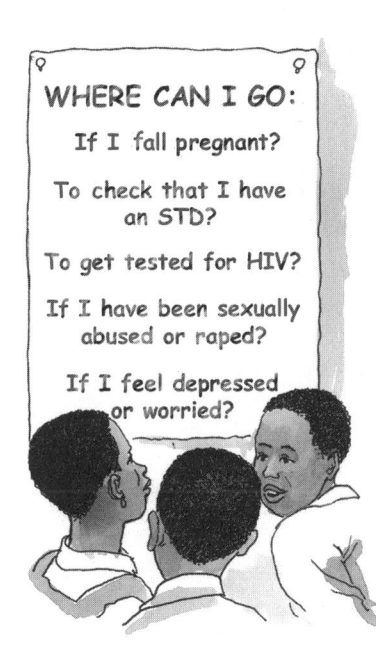

Ideas for the classroom

Older primary school children need to know about the signs of STDs (see opposite page) and what to do about them. After you have given them the information you can play this game, which helps to reinforce the fact that HIV and AIDS together are an STD, and reinforces the ABCD of protection:

1. One child stands in the middle of a circle of seven other children. She or he is called the STD Protector.
2. Each of the other seven children is given a piece of paper with the one following messages on it: 'Abstains from sex.' 'Is faithful to a tested partner.' 'Uses condoms.' 'Has many sexual partners.' 'Doesn't know how to say NO to sex.' 'Refuses to wear condoms.' 'Likes to date people who are a lot older'.

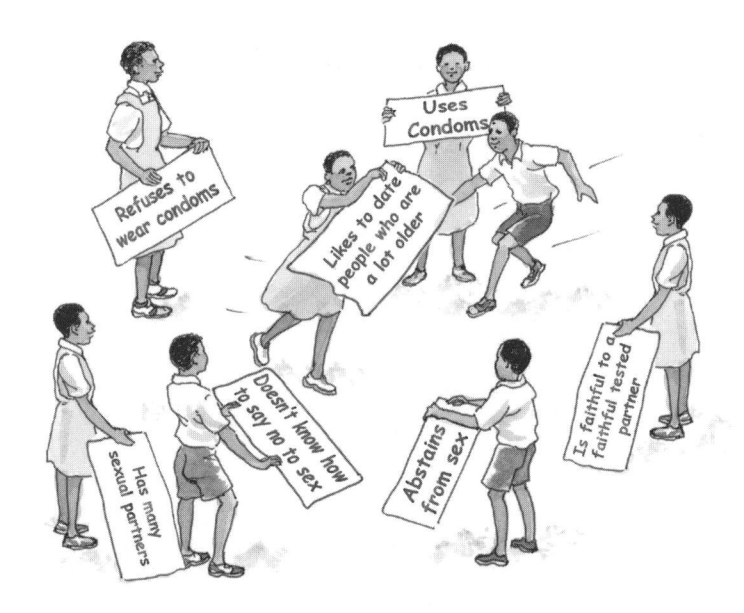

3. These children run across and the Protector tries to catch one child. When they are caught they have to read their paper and say whether their behaviour puts them in danger of getting an STD. Ask the rest of the class whether they agree. The children who, according to the rest of the class, are not safe, are out of the game.
4. Once the children have understood the game you could give the ones who are out another chance to write a statement which is 'safe' and join the game again. The class then has to decide if they agree that person is really safe form catching STDs. The point of the game is to get discussions about safe behaviour going.

This game is an adaptation of an original version that appeared in an extract from *Participatory Package and Quality Assurance*, © D Wilson and R Kathuria, Lusaka, Zambia, and published in *Happy, Healthy and Safe: Youth-to-youth learning activities on growing up, relationships, sexual health, HIV/AIDS, life skills*, compiled and edited by Andrew Hobbs et al, Family Health Trust (Anti-AIDS project) Lusaka, Zambia, 1988

WHERE CAN I GO:

If I fall pregnant?

To check that I have an STD?

To get tested for HIV?

If I have been sexually abused or raped?

If I feel depressed or worried?

Activity *Let children know where they can get help*

Make sure that the children, however young they are, know where to get help with sexual health. Make a list of these places. You can put the information in a place where they can look at it without feeling ashamed. You could even ask the children to help you find this information.

Helpful hint

When teaching about STDs, make sure that children do not associate them with shame or pride. Some children can get an STD because they were abused, and need support rather than judgement.

40 Sex and power

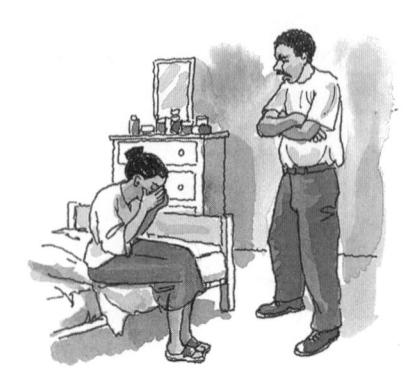

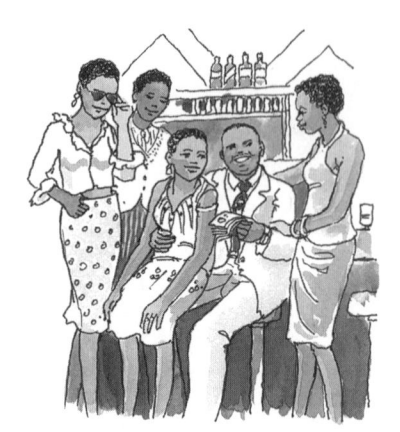

Bullying and sex

Sometimes, people have sex because they want to show they have power over one another. For example, a husband can have sex with his wife to show her that he is in charge. A headmaster could have sex with a teacher to show that he is boss. Sex can be used to bully another person.

Activity   Gender roles

Think about your community. Are there any situations where sex is used to show power over others?

In most societies, men have far more power than women. This is because of the roles that our cultures have given to men and women. We call them gender roles. This table shows some beliefs about gender roles.

Males should	Females should
Be in control and dominate women.	Be submissive and obey men.
Have sex with many partners.	Remain virgins for as long as possible.
Drink alcohol.	Be sober and sensible.
Put their own needs first.	Put the needs of others first.
Take risks and be aggressive.	Be soft and unassertive.

Can you think of more examples?

These roles may seem natural but they were created by people. Gender roles can put both males and females at risk of getting infected with HIV.

Case study

This story shows how girls and boys often have sex without discussing it and without protection, because of gender roles. Do you think it could happen in your community?

This case study explains how gender roles can put people in danger.

May is 13 and Joseph is 15. They are very sad. They have just had sex for the first time. They like each other very much and have known each other since they were children. They did not enjoy having sex, but Joseph felt that he had to. He did not want May to think that he was weak. His friend, Ben, had been teasing him for a long time.

'I have already been with four girls and you are still a virgin,' Ben had said. 'What kind of a man are you?'

Joseph decided that he would have sex with May. He could see that she did not want to, and it made him unhappy.

May could not say 'No' because she felt that, as a girl, she could not argue with a boy.

Joseph had sex with her because he did not want her to think he was weak.

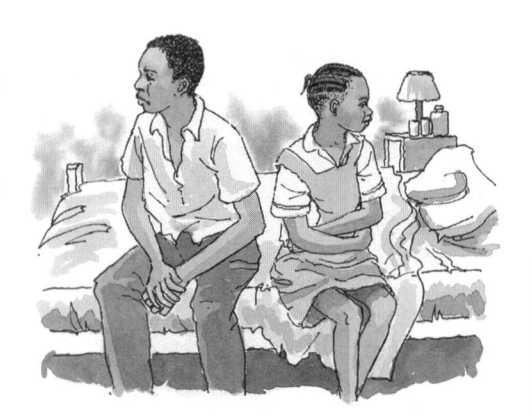

Sex and sexuality

Did you know?

In Africa and many other regions, young women are more exposed to AIDS than young men. Here are some reasons for this.

Traditionally, they have sex with older, more experienced men. Many men are looking for even younger women to have sex with because of HIV and AIDS. They think that young girls, especially virgins, will be free from HIV.

Many women are completely dependent on their husbands or partners for money and support. This can make it difficult for them to refuse sex or to insist that a condom is used.

In some societies, it is acceptable for men to be violent towards their wives or partners. This makes it harder to refuse sex. In many countries, there are no laws against a husband raping his wife.

Men sometimes feel that it is their right to have more than one sexual partner.

Ideas for the classroom

It is important that boys and girls are aware of gender roles and how these can lead to risky situations. Show them the picture of May and Joseph and ask what they think has happened, and why. The information in the 'Did you know?' box may help them think of ideas.

Divide the class into groups – some of boys and some of girls.

The girls discuss what it is like to be a girl – what makes it hard and what makes it easy? Boys discuss what it is like to be a boy – what makes it hard and what makes it easy?

Then, in groups of four, let two girls talk to two boys about what it is like to be a girl. Next, the boys talk to the girls about what it is like to be a boy.

Let the groups discuss how men and women in your community see each other. Are they equal? What negative feelings do they have towards each other? What positive feelings do they have?

Help boys and girls think about the fact that many girls are taught to be submissive to men and that this makes them more vulnerable to HIV infection.

Allow a few pairs to report back to the whole class.

Ask every group to describe the kinds of experiences that make it easy for them to get HIV.

Towards the end the lesson, talk about what can make gender roles dangerous and how they can help spread HIV and AIDS. Ask the class to draw up a list of actions that can help them to be more respectful to each other. For example, boys and girls will listen to each other. When a girl says 'No!' to sex a boy will take her seriously. (See also Topic 29, page 62.)

Encourage boys to think about how they take risks of getting HIV for the sake of proving their manhood.

Encourage the girls to think about how relationships put them at risk.

Talk about the case study to start a class discussion about how to make the world a safer place for young people, especially girls.

Helpful hints

- Be clear. Think about the abuse of power in relationships and decide where you stand.
- Be critical. Do not apologise for harmful or irresponsible behaviour, even if it is traditional or widespread.
- Be positive. Encourage young people to make a difference and to build a better world. (See also Section 3, pages 38–67.)

Section 5 Teaching about HIV in all areas of the curriculum

41 When and how to teach about HIV

> *Definition*
>
> A **curriculum** tells you about the courses that are offered at a school – what is taught, how it is taught, why it is taught.

Three ways to teach about HIV and AIDS

There are three basic ways in which teaching about HIV and AIDS can become part of the school curriculum. The first way is to introduce a separate course about HIV and AIDS. The second way is to use part of the existing curriculum, such as a Life Skills programme or science lessons, and to teach lessons about how HIV is spread and about how to care for people living with AIDS. The third way is to teach about HIV and AIDS across the curriculum, in every subject, wherever it will fit in.

Activity The best way to teach about HIV

Think about how best to teach about HIV/AIDS at school. How would you do it? Why?

Now look at the three models below. Discuss the advantages and disadvantages of each model.

Model 1

Teach a separate course that focuses only on HIV and AIDS

The good thing about teaching a separate course about HIV and AIDS is that your teaching is very focused and you are telling people it is very important.

One problem with this approach is that it will give children information, but information alone does not change behaviour. What else do you need?

Model 2

Teach about HIV and AIDS as part of the Life Skills curriculum

A lot of information about HIV links to general Life Skills (see Topic 47, pages 100–101). When we talk about universal precautions, for example, we also have to talk about First Aid. When we talk about how HIV is spread, we have to talk about sex. That is why it makes sense to teach about HIV and AIDS as part of the general Life Skills curriculum. Here, the teacher not only focuses on passing on information, but also on developing skills.

A disadvantage of doing this, however, is that the curriculum is very full, and this leaves too little time to give HIV and AIDS the attention they deserve.

Model 3

Teach about HIV and AIDS as part of the whole curriculum

It is a good idea for all teachers to focus on HIV and AIDS in their classes, as it affects all parts of life. When HIV and AIDS is mentioned again and again, the children will realise that it is a serious issue and they will slowly build up a good understanding of the epidemic and how it affects people's relationships and their health. One problem is that not every teacher will co-operate with this approach. Another problem is that children may get bored with too much talk about HIV and AIDS.

Teaching about HIV in all areas of the curriculum

Activity *Identifying factors that will lead to a successful programme*

Most teachers do not have a choice about where and when to teach about HIV. Sometimes the syllabus, the school principal or government guidelines tell teachers what to do. Even if teachers have no choice about what to teach, they can still think about how to do it.

- Which factors will help any HIV programme to succeed?

> honesty
> good knowledge
> caring
> listening to questions
> involving young people
> confidence
> ....
> ....
> ....
> ....

Perhaps the best way to teach about HIV and AIDS is to use more than one approach. A mix of models will give the children good background knowledge about HIV and AIDS and allow enough time for developing Life Skills that change attitudes and behaviours. A mix of methods (stories, role-play, art, lessons, exercises) also helps all children to get involved.

Case study

When the teachers of Jabula Primary School decided to talk about HIV and AIDS to their children, they decided to run an HIV and AIDS campaign for one term.

First, they sent one teacher for training. The job of this teacher was to learn how to offer a course about HIV and AIDS to both the children and parents of the school.

The courses for children and adults were presented separately after school hours. Everyone who was interested could attend.

While these courses were going on, the other teachers also helped to make HIV and AIDS part of the general curriculum of the school.

- The Art teacher ran an art competition for the best poster about preventing HIV.
- The Science teacher planned a lesson on germs and talked about HIV.
- The Social Studies teacher asked the children to write about the way they were going to avoid HIV infections in the future.
- The English teacher asked the children to write stories about the way HIV and AIDS were affecting their lives.

In this way, they all worked together to get the school community involved.

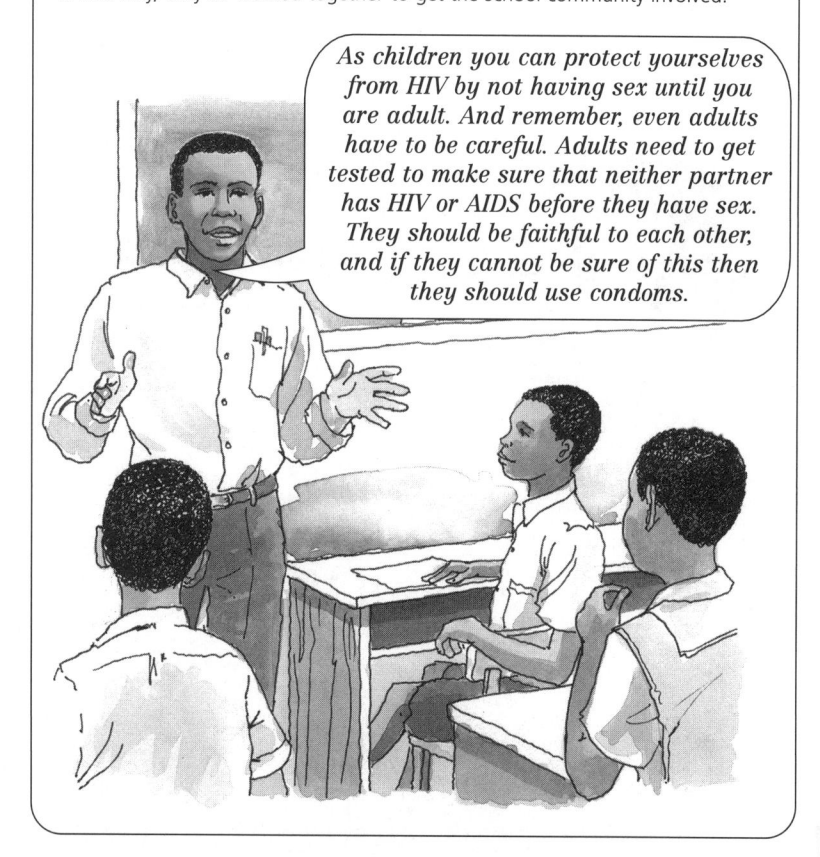

As children you can protect yourselves from HIV by not having sex until you are adult. And remember, even adults have to be careful. Adults need to get tested to make sure that neither partner has HIV or AIDS before they have sex. They should be faithful to each other, and if they cannot be sure of this then they should use condoms.

42 Teaching about HIV and AIDS in all subject areas

Definition
A **concept** is a key idea that helps us to make sense of other information and ideas. Concepts help to organise our particular experiences and ideas into a more general understanding of the world.

HIV and AIDS and the curriculum

In most countries, the primary school curriculum was fixed long before HIV and AIDS were seen as important topics to teach about. Teachers who are committed to helping children understand more about HIV and AIDS often have to fit these lessons in with other subjects.

For example, you have seen in previous sections that HIV is a biological and medical problem. There is a clear link between understanding HIV and understanding how diseases work. We can, therefore, use the biology and science curriculum to develop the basic concepts that can help children to understand HIV.

Activity 1 Linking what you teach with HIV and AIDS

Make a list of the subjects you are expected to teach. Think about how each of these subjects gives you an opportunity to help children understand HIV and AIDS.

How can we educate children about HIV if we do not teach them what a germ is? Even if the lesson on germs does not mention AIDS, the concept that germs cause diseases is an important mental building block for all children. Without it they will never really understand how HIV works.

Even teaching History is useful. When we teach our children about the slave trade, we are teaching about a time when millions of people were moved from one continent to another area of the world. This changed the way societies worked in both places. By asking good questions about the slave trade – for example, its effects on family relationships and society, and the importance of maintaining self-respect – the children gain the mental tools for thinking about how HIV can affect people's lives.

Why did it happen? What do you think is risky about this? What does this remind you of?

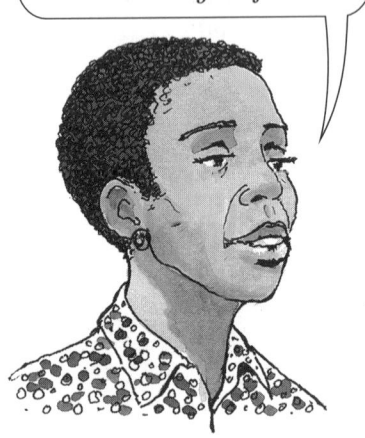

Ask open questions to encourage discussion.

Activity 2 Examine the syllabus

Go to your syllabus and look through the content of the subjects you teach. Make a list of all the topics and concepts that can be 'mental building blocks' for understanding HIV and AIDS. Also, refer to your syllabus on HIV and AIDS education if there is one. Here is an example:

Subject	Concept	Building block
Health	Reproduction	Understanding reproduction is a building block for understanding how having sex can spread HIV (link to HIV and AIDS).
Maths	Multiplication	Understanding multiplication is a building block for understanding why HIV is spreading very quickly when people have more than one sexual partner.

Build teaching about HIV and AIDS into your schemes of work. Share ideas with your colleagues and decide how to deal with overlaps from one subject to another.

Teaching about HIV in all areas of the curriculum

Here is another way to help you to think about teaching HIV and AIDS across the curriculum. You can treat teaching about HIV as an investigation.

Step 1: Identify the problem under investigation

For example, how do we grow up, have babies and have families without getting HIV?

Step 2: What knowledge do children need about HIV?

Identify the mental building blocks for this investigation and teach them. For example, do the children have accurate information about reproduction? Do they know how HIV is spread? Do they know about condoms and how they work? Do they know about HIV testing?

Step 3: What skills do they need? What values do they need to solve the problem under investigation?

For example, do the children know how to be boyfriends or girlfriends without having sex? Are they confident enough to say 'No'? Are they comfortable talking about sex? Do they accept people living with HIV? Do they know how to go for an HIV test?

Step 5: What will the outcome of the investigation be?

How will the children present their work? For example, will the children write a paragraph about how they can start their own family without HIV? Will they present a speech?

Step 4: How much time do you need for this investigation?

For example, do you need time to teach the basic information first, before you start the investigation? How many lessons do you need for group work?

Helpful hints

Use questions to help learners make the connections between subject knowledge and HIV.

For example, if you teach the class about a healthy diet, ask the children which foods help to keep the body healthy (A: fruit, vegetables, especially greens).

Then ask them which part of the body is most affected when you have HIV (A: the immune system).

Finally, ask them which foods would be good for a person living with HIV (A: fruit, vegetables, especially greens).

Activity   Teaching as an investigation

Think about teaching as an investigation of a problem. What do you like about this approach? What do you not like? Why?

Remember

- Don't preach about HIV and AIDS. Investigate them!

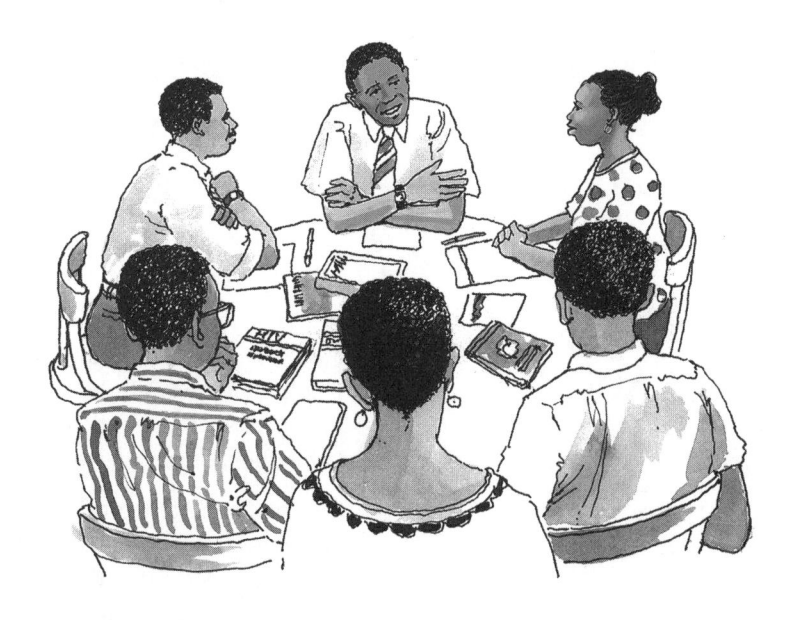

43 Using science lessons to teach about HIV and AIDS

Definition

A **project** is a long task set on a specific topic. It encourages pupils to find out information on their own and to present it in a creative way.

'**Contextualising**' knowledge means taking a general idea and thinking how it would apply to a particular situation or context.

HIV and AIDS as a context

Science, health or biology lessons offer many good opportunities to talk to children about what HIV is and how it is spread.

If you teach these subjects, you can use HIV as an example for the concept you are trying to teach. In other words, you can contextualise the scientific concepts in terms of HIV and AIDS. If you teach about germs, use HIV to give an example of a germ. If you teach about how babies are born, mention mother-to-child transmission of HIV. (See Topic 38, pages 80–83.) If you teach about epidemics, you can use HIV as an example of a new infection that has taken the world by surprise.

Scientific knowledge

Good scientific knowledge of HIV and AIDS is important. It helps young people to understand what is happening around them and gives them a solid foundation of facts about the disease. This can help them to cope when members of their families fall ill. Those who understand how HIV multiplies and spreads will also find it easier to challenge wrong information about condoms, sex and HIV.

Activity   Look at the science curriculum

Look at the science curriculum for your school. Which lessons in the curriculum allow you to talk about HIV and how it is spread? How would you fit the following lessons into the existing curriculum?

- HIV is a sexually transmitted disease.
- Babies can become infected with HIV during pregnancy or birth.
- You can protect yourself from HIV if you do not have sex or delay sex for as long as possible.
- Test yourself and your partner for HIV before you have sex.
- Use a condom to prevent the spread of HIV.

Health workers

Ask your local health workers to help you teach about HIV and AIDS. Many are trained to talk openly about sexuality or reproductive health and know all the facts. They can talk about prevention methods, such as condoms, from a medical point of view and often know the kinds of questions young people have.

This helps them to give good advice about preventing HIV. Another advantage of inviting a local health worker is that it introduces medical personnel to the school and the health needs of the pupils. Young people get a chance to meet the staff at their local clinic and this makes it easier to go there when they need help.

Teaching about HIV in all areas of the curriculum

Some teachers plan projects specifically on HIV and AIDS. Although project work needs more planning than usual and uses more time, it gives children an opportunity to investigate the epidemic in the context of their own lives. A well-planned project can empower children to think about information on their own. It also encourages them to ask questions.

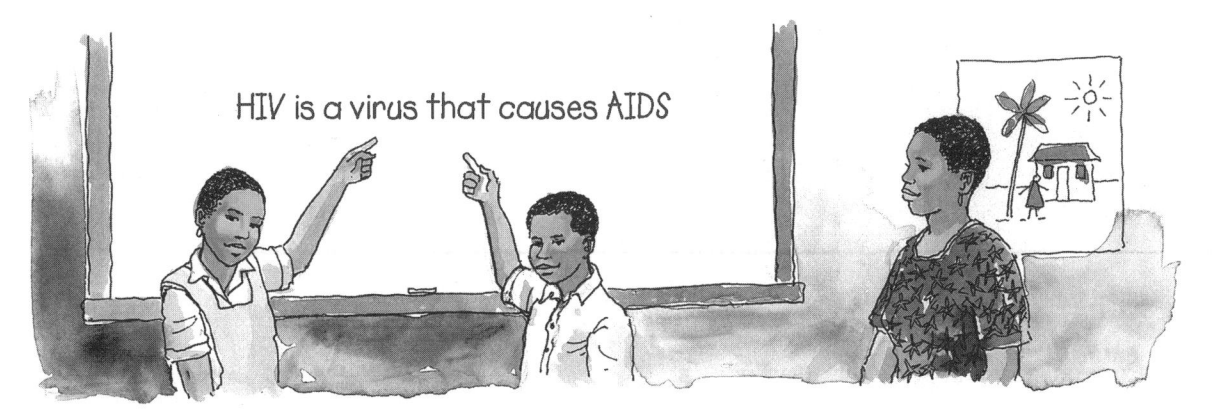

HIV is a virus that causes AIDS

The illustration shows two pupils presenting their own science lesson, sharing what they have learnt about HIV. The teacher is listening carefully to make sure that all the information they present is correct. After the presentation, she or he should encourage the pupils to investigate the topic further so they can see the value of this knowledge for their lives.

Here are some useful questions to ask.

- How would you use this information when you decide to start a family?
- Who would be a good person to choose as husband or wife?
- What should you discuss with your partner before having sex?
- Where could you go for a HIV test?
- Where can you get counselling or advice?

Activity Look for links

Notice how all the questions on the right create a link between the general information about HIV and the real life challenges young people face. What other questions could you ask?

Ideas for the classroom

Prepare a short general quiz about HIV and AIDS to find out what your pupils already know about HIV and AIDS. Here are some sample questions:

1. What is HIV?
2. Which part of the body is affected by HIV infections?
3. Why is it a serious disease?
4. Name three ways in which HIV is spread.
5. Name three ways in which you can protect yourself from the disease.

The answers to this quiz are found on page 131.

The result of the quiz can guide you in your planning. What basic information is missing? Do all children know how and why sex can infect them with HIV?

Helpful hints

- Ask interesting questions about HIV.
- Use your science lesson to make links to HIV, when the lesson provides the children with a key concept for understanding HIV and AIDS.
- Answer all questions honestly and openly, even if they make you feel a little uncomfortable.

44 Using stories and readers to teach about HIV and AIDS

The importance of stories

We all love a good story. Throughout the ages, stories have been used as very powerful teaching tools.

Africa, in particular, has a very strong story-telling tradition. Grandmothers use myths and animal tales to teach children right from wrong. Praise poets recite long poems to teach the history of the clan. Teachers can use their narrative heritage to teach children about HIV and AIDS. Stories help to make HIV and AIDS education more effective. Here are a few reasons why this is so.

- Stories engage the head and the heart.
- Stories can help us to think about something in the context of a real life situation. They capture complexity.
- Stories go beyond the boundaries of here and now. They link the past and the future. They can bring the whole world into the class.
- Stories give us 'plots' to help make sense of the big questions in life. They also model good choices and teach children how to be honest, caring or brave.
- Stories give everyone the opportunity to imagine new endings for old problems. With the help of stories, we can 'rewrite' our life.

Activity The story of Jacob

Here is the beginning of Jacob's story. Jacob lives in a family affected by AIDS.

Jacob is on his way to school. His school is far away and Jacob is feeling very hungry. His legs are weak. He feels very alone. How will he ever get to school on time?

Suddenly he notices an old woman sitting on a stone next to the road. As he comes closer, she …

What happened next? Make up your own ending in three different ways.

- Ending 1: Jacob is the victim of the situation.
- Ending 2: Jacob is the hero of the moment.
- Ending 3: Jacob cannot solve the problem on his own, but gets help.

Which ending did you like best? Why?

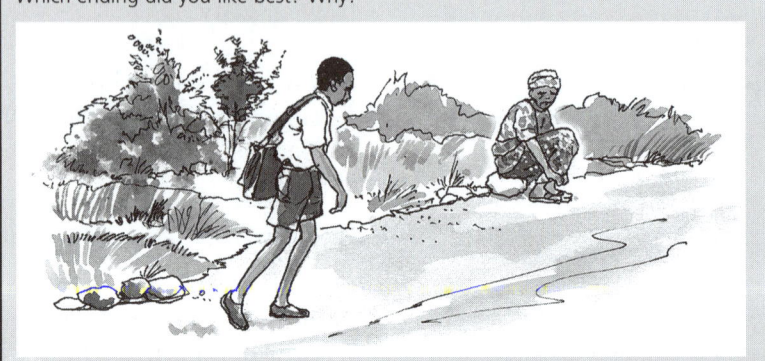

Teaching about HIV in all areas of the curriculum

There are many different possibilities for using stories and readers to teach about HIV or AIDS. Here are a few ideas:

1 Read stories to give courage and hope.
- Read stories to the class for enjoyment.
- Choose stories that express emotion.
- Choose stories that show people doing the right thing.
- Do not 'work' with the story too much. Allow it to be simply a good story that gives hope.

2 Read stories to model behaviour change.
- Allow children to read stories alone, or read to them.
- Choose stories that show how behaviour changed and why. For example, a story about a girl who begins to wear gloves when touching blood.

Talk about people's behaviour in the story. Ask questions like, 'Why is she behaving like this?' 'What does she get out of being like this?' 'Could she have done it differently?' 'How? What changed?' 'Why?' 'Is it a change for the better?'

3 Read stories to give more detailed information.
- Allow children to read these stories several times so they become familiar with the content.
- Choose stories that give simple but accurate information. For example, read a story about a boy who accompanies his mother, when she goes for HIV testing.
- Talk about the information in the story. Ask questions that help to clarify the content, such as, 'What happens when you go for testing?' 'What is tested?' 'When will she have the result?' 'How does she feel?'

4 Read stories to create a talking point about choices.
- Read a story to the children and allow them to enjoy it. Encourage the children to put themselves into the story.

Choose stories that have a central problem or dilemma that has to be solved. You can also use letters that are seeking advice. Talk about the problem to explore it from all sides. Talk about possible solutions and make sure that the message about safe choices is very clear.

Tell children, the best protection from HIV is to not have sex, to do an HIV test with their partner before they start having sex, and to use a condom.

Helpful hints
- Don't rush with stories. Allow enough time for reading and talking.
- Readers and stories are not only part of language teaching. All of the methods described in this topic can be used in subject teaching as well.

Activity Think about your use of stories
How have you used stories in your teaching?
Which of the possibilities suggested in this topic do you find most helpful? Why?

45 Using Social Studies lessons to teach about HIV and AIDS

Definition

Social Studies includes Environmental and Social Studies and subjects such as History, Geography or Civics.

Activity **Planning the curriculum**

Think about way to fit the topics listed on the right into your existing curriculum.

- What HIV and AIDS teaching is required in your Social Studies curriculum?
- What other interesting links can you see between your Social Studies curriculum and HIV and AIDS? Try to think of at least three.

The study of people

All the subjects in the Social Studies curriculum have one thing in common: they all study people.

In History, we explore how people and nations have developed, what conflicts they had and how these were resolved. In Geography or Environmental Studies, we look at where people live and how they live. With its focus on society and people, the Social Studies curriculum therefore gives teachers many opportunities to teach about HIV and AIDS. Often Social Studies syllabuses include Health Education, Life Skills and HIV and AIDS education.

Here are some interesting topics for investigation.

- Why AIDS is a new disease.
- The traditional roles of men, women and children, and how these are changing when a community is affected by HIV and AIDS.
- The social conditions that help HIV to spread quickly.
- How to start healthy families in a community affected by HIV and AIDS.

The Social Studies curriculum

The Social Studies curriculum already helps young people to understand the implications of HIV and AIDS on their lives.

It teaches about ideas such as:

- Crisis
- Social and personal implications of an event
- Social change

It also teaches important values such as:

- Making a difference
- Equality
- Justice
- Democracy

It encourages skills such as:

- Decision-making
- Problem-solving
- Listening
- Having an opinion

The biggest advantage of using Social Studies lessons to teach about HIV and AIDS is that they can encourage pupils to look at the implications of HIV and AIDS for their own lives.

'If–then'

With a simple technique like the 'if–then' investigation, teachers can help children to think deeply about the society of which they are part. The following steps outline the process of making up an 'if–then' thinking chain that is at the heart of the investigation. By presenting the two words, 'if' and 'then', teachers are helping pupils to look for the impact or consequences of one thing for another. For example:

- *If* you sleep late *then* you will be late for school.
- *If* you do not eat breakfast *then* you will be hungry at school.

Teaching about HIV in all areas of the curriculum

Here is an example of an 'if-then' investigation about the impact of HIV on families. With a little help, children can learn to follow these steps for themselves at primary school.

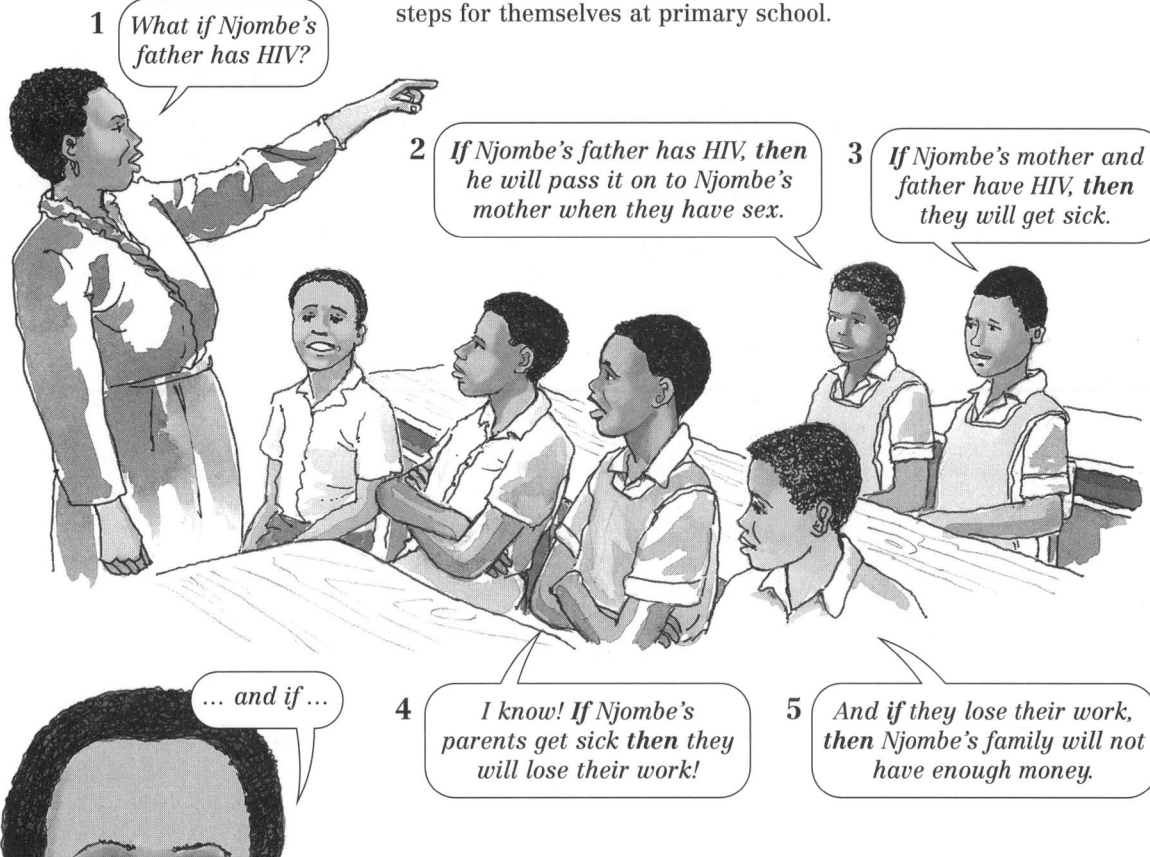

1 *What if Njombe's father has HIV?*

2 *If Njombe's father has HIV, then he will pass it on to Njombe's mother when they have sex.*

3 *If Njombe's mother and father have HIV, then they will get sick.*

... and if ...

4 *I know! If Njombe's parents get sick then they will lose their work!*

5 *And if they lose their work, then Njombe's family will not have enough money.*

The success of a 'if–then' investigation depends on three things:

- The teacher must ask a clear, but thought-provoking question at the beginning.
- The teacher must be strict about the way the pupils respond. Only 'if–then' sentences are allowed.

The teacher must challenge any if–then sentences that are too vague or do not really show consequence. For example, 'if Njombe's father has HIV, then it will be bad' is not a good reply. The teacher can challenge this reply by asking, 'What will be bad? What exactly will happen?'

Helpful hints

- Use the steps suggested in this topic as a model for teaching pupils to investigate ideas.
- Choose only one question for each investigation.
- Listen to the children and encourage the children to think on their own.
- Do not insist on only one 'correct' answer. There are many ways in which HIV affects our lives. Your job is to make sure the 'if–then' relationship is accurate and clear.

Activity   Your own investigation

Make up your own if–then investigation, starting with the question 'What if teachers refuse to teach about HIV?'

Here are some more questions to try.

- Sipho is HIV positive. What if Sipho asks his girlfriend to have sex with him?
- What if Sipho's girlfriend refuses?
- What if she agrees?

46 Linking your teaching about HIV and AIDS to life

HIV and the children's experience

Teaching about HIV is not the same as teaching other subjects in the curriculum. It is not an abstract topic and should not be separated from the experiences of the children in class.

Children may remember very little HIV information if it is not relevant to their lives. They do not listen if HIV and AIDS are simply added onto the lesson like a slogan and is repeated over and over again. They will, however, pay attention if talking about HIV helps them to explore and answer real questions and problems they might have.

Personal experience can be a very powerful teaching tool in the fight against HIV and AIDS. When teachers link their lessons to the experiences of children in their class, the lessons usually become more interesting and easier to understand.

Children quickly become personally involved and find it easier to share their ideas. They also feel the lessons are important because they deal with real problems and real solutions.

This table contains six questions that can help you to link your lessons about HIV to the lives of the children in your class.

> *Activity* Complete these sentences
>
> My pupils seem most interested when ...
> My pupils get bored when ...
> My pupils feel something is important to them when ...
> My pupils care mostly about ...

What do the children already know from experience?	What strong feelings might they have about this topic?	What teaching points will help them to avoid getting HIV?
What about HIV or AIDS will interest them the most?	What method can I use to help them share their experiences and ideas about the topic?	What activities will help them to practise the skills they need to avoid HIV infection?

> *Activity* More questions to think about
>
> Think about these questions, too.
> - How can the children's personal experiences help in teaching about HIV and AIDS?
> - What about those who have cared for a sick relatives, or who know of someone who has a positive attitude to living with HIV?
> - What kinds of experiences would be difficult to deal with in class?
>   How would you respond to experiences of rape or abuse?
> - What kinds of experiences need to be treated with sensitivity and care? For example, how would you talk about having HIV in the family? How would you talk about death?

Teaching about HIV in all areas of the curriculum

Talking about HIV in a personalised way

Talking about HIV in a personalised way, however, is never easy. It quickly brings out strong feelings and opinions, but also many questions and fears.

Children often do not want to share their personal experiences because this is painful or because they are afraid others will laugh at them. Teachers are reluctant to share their personal experiences because they worry about their reputation and about gossip in the school.

Case studies and role-plays are useful methods that bring a personal perspective to your teaching, without forcing your pupils to share experiences that are too painful for them.

> **Activity** *Your own case study*
>
> Read the case study on this page and then write your own case study to help you to teach about HIV in your community.

> ### Helpful hints
>
> If you are using the case study about Jamima in class, make sure all the children understand the story.
>
> Ask questions that help them think about Jamima's problem. Here are a few examples.
> - What if Jamima refuses to have sex with her uncle?
> - What if Jamima runs away?
> - What if Jamima has sex with him?
> - How can Jamima protect herself from HIV?
> - Who can Jamima ask for help with this problem?
> - Who can tell the uncle that it is against the law to have sex with children?

> ### Case study
>
> Jamima is a bright girl. She loves going to school. But it is difficult for her, because her family is poor.
>
> When her father died, Jamima was sent to live at her uncle's home.
>
> At first, she was happy, because her uncle is rich. He promised to pay her school fees.
>
> But now she has a problem. Her uncle wants to have sex with her, in return for the money he pays for her fees.
>
> She is too young for sex, and she is afraid of HIV.
> - Can she refuse him?
> - What should she do?

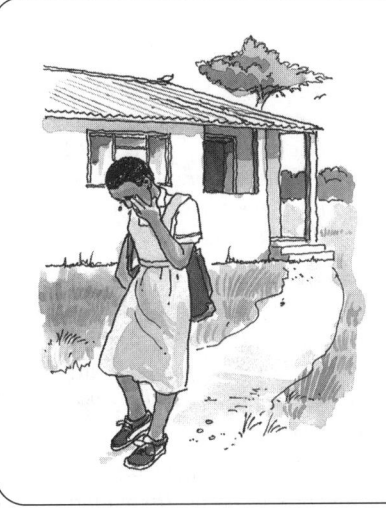

47 Teaching Life Skills at school

Making Life Skills a formal part of the curriculum

Life Skills education has been happening in the family and in the community for many generations. As children grew up, their parents and caregivers encouraged them to develop those skills and attitudes that would help the children to become independent and cope with the problems they might face. Teaching children to look after their personal needs was part of the informal curriculum and did not directly affect what a teacher would do in class.

In the past ten years, there has been a change. More and more schools are making Life Skills a formal part of their curriculum and use class time to nurture the personal and social skills that will help young people to operate effectively in society once they leave school.

Some teachers welcome this change, others are critical of it, saying that parents are the primary educators of their children and schools should not be expected to do their job.

Different kinds of Life Skills

Life Skills are about personal skills, such as self-awareness, confidence, problem-solving and coping with emotion. Inter-personal Life Skills are about good communication, assertiveness and working together. Life skills may also be about practical skills, such as cooking or managing money.

Definition

Life Skills are abilities which help us to adapt and to behave positively so that we can deal effectively with the challenges of everyday life.

Life Skills include: decision-making; interpersonal skills; critical thinking; negotiation; resistance; problem-solving; empathy; creative thinking; communication; goal-setting; self awareness; assertiveness; coping.

Activity Thinking about your own Life Skills

Talk about some of the skills and attitudes your family taught you. What has been the most valuable lesson that helped you cope with life? For example, it might be to try to change those things you can change and accept those things you can't.

What do you personally think about teaching Life Skills in school?

Give reasons for your answer.

At first I was very critical of teaching Life Skills. I thought that it is not part of my job. Children should be taught at home how to look after their personal needs. In the last two years, I have changed my mind. I can see how AIDS is breaking families apart. So it is better we teach the children what they need to know at school.

With AIDS, children are growing up too soon. Children are working and looking after their parents long before they are grown. This makes them independent. But it also gives them emotional problems that we have not had in our community before. So the traditional Life Skills education in the family is not always effective.

I believe it is part of my responsibility to make sure our children can survive if they happen to be on their own.

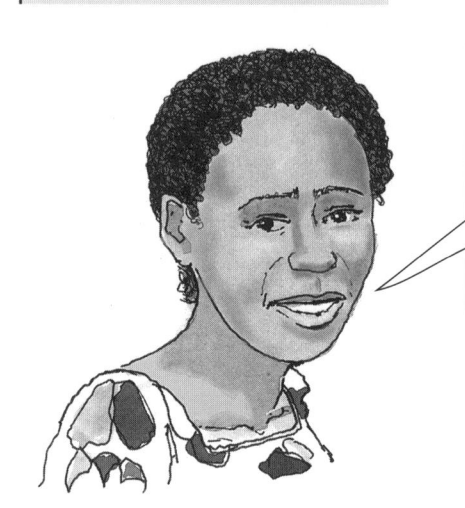

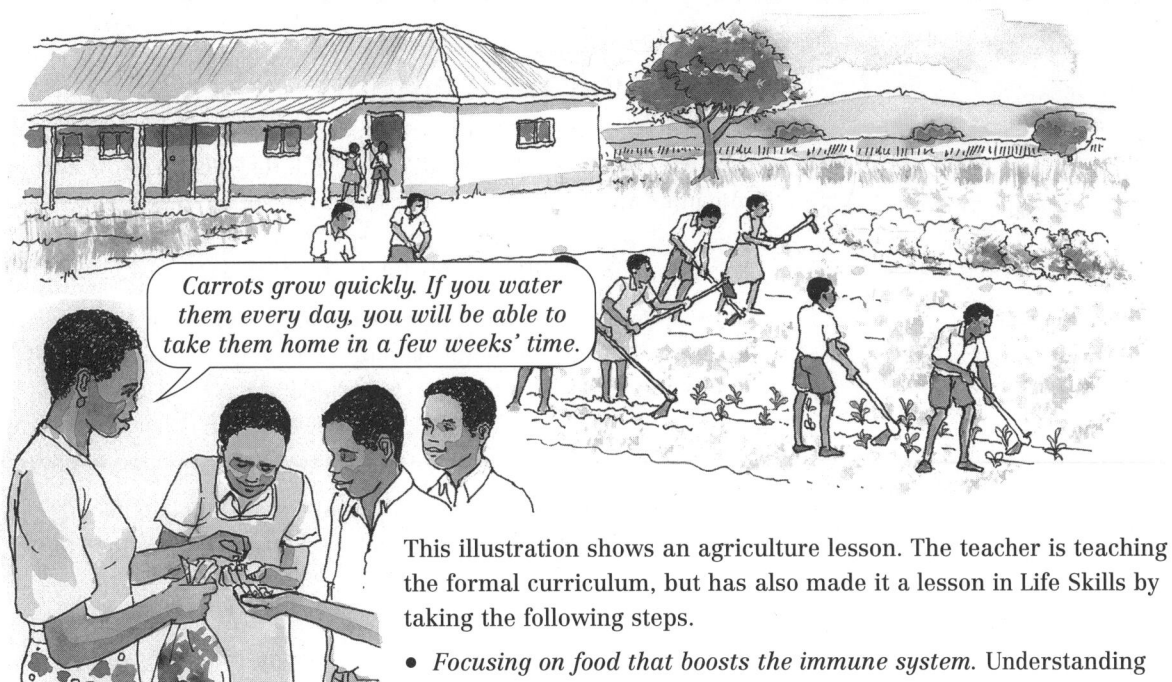

Teaching about HIV in all areas of the curriculum

Carrots grow quickly. If you water them every day, you will be able to take them home in a few weeks' time.

This illustration shows an agriculture lesson. The teacher is teaching the formal curriculum, but has also made it a lesson in Life Skills by taking the following steps.

- *Focusing on food that boosts the immune system.* Understanding what food is good for the immune system is important knowledge for children whose parents are ill.
- *Being practical.* She is not only giving children the information, but is also teaching them how to grow nutritious food. Getting cheap, but healthy meals is an important skill for children affected by HIV.
- *Being gender-sensitive and promoting gender fairness.* She is expecting both boys and girls to dig and grow food. In this way she is nurturing new values that help to fight HIV.
- *Involving everybody.* All children are active and this helps to make learning more meaningful for them.
- *Growing food for children.* She is sensitive to the lived experience of HIV. Her school is in a poor community, and many children are probably hungry when they come to school. Through this lesson, she is not only giving them information, but is also showing care and compassion. These are important values in a society affected by AIDS.

Ideas for the classroom

Extend the above lesson by helping the children to draw up a cheap, nutritious menu for a person living with HIV.

The children should copy a list of 'good foods' in their notebooks. They can also make up a song to remember food that is good for the immune system. They can then sing it to their parents at home.

Some schools have started school gardens to support children who care for sick adults at home.

Activity   The lesson in the picture

What do you think of the lesson shown in the picture? How practical is it? How would you go about teaching a lesson like this?

Helpful hints

You can help to make teaching Life Skills meaningful by:
- taking a personal interest in the lives of the children and noticing how HIV and AIDS affect them
- responding honestly to the questions children ask
- having the courage to say, 'I don't know. Let's find this out together.'

48 Teaching effective communication

Definitions

Effective communication is the ability to express your ideas clearly and to exchange ideas with others.

Empathy is the ability to understand other people's feelings.

Activity Questions to think about

Are you an effective communicator? What makes you effective? What makes it difficult for you to express and share your ideas?

Communication and HIV

Effective communication is very important in the fight against HIV. How can young people abstain from sex if they do not know how to communicate their ideas? How can they negotiate new kinds of relationships if they are too shy to speak? How will they learn to respect each other if they only think of themselves?

Every lesson in every subject can be an opportunity for teachers to encourage effective communication. It happens when teachers allow children to express their ideas. It happens when children work in groups and listen to each other. It happens when teachers encourage children to ask questions and allow differences in opinion to exist.

There are two skills that make children confident when they communicate with others. These are self-awareness and empathy.

Self-awareness

I know myself. I am happy to be alive. I know what I feel and what I want from life. I accept my character and know what I am good at, but also what my weaknesses are. I think about what is happening around me and this helps me to decide what is best for me.

Empathy

I try to understand others, especially if they are different from me. I imagine what life is like for them. I wonder what I would feel if I were in their place. I also look at people's faces when I talk to them. It helps me to know how they are feeling. Are they happy? Are they sad? How can I reach out to them?

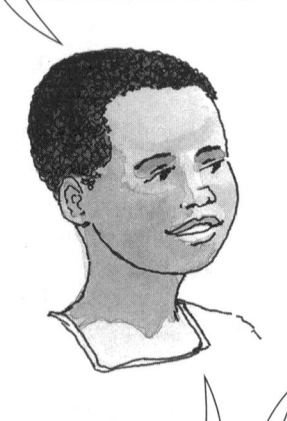

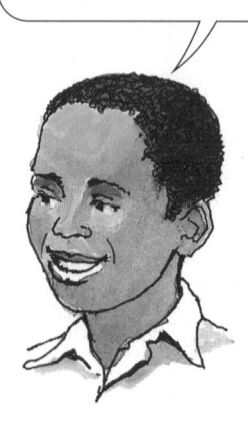

Effective communication

If I am aware of who I am and what I like, it is easier to express my thoughts and share my ideas. If I do not have empathy, I might say things that are selfish or hurtful to others. Empathy helps me connect with others and get my message across. It also helps me to listen and to respect other people's ideas.

Teaching about HIV in all areas of the curriculum

The illustration shows that effective communication is both internal and external. The internal processes of self-awareness and empathy are the foundations for the external exchange of ideas.

Both the internal and external parts of effective communication can be nurtured through the way you teach about HIV and AIDS.

> ### Activity   Plan a lesson
> Plan a lesson on how HIV is spread. Make sure your lesson includes one exercise that will help the children become aware of their own feelings about HIV. Include a second exercise that encourages children to think about the feelings of others.

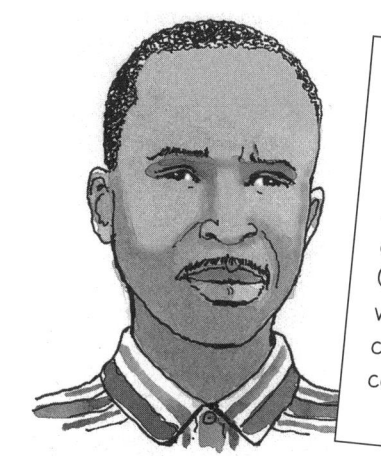

Mr Okello writes:

Many of my pupils are too shy to speak up when I ask them a question in class. They seem to have no opinions and no ideas. Class discussions are a waste of time. How can I help them to communicate?

What can Mr Okello do?

Mr Okello could try asking a question and then giving the children two minutes to whisper among themselves, telling each other what they think the answer could be. Then he can ask for a volunteer to answer the question.

Once he has heard the answer, he can ask the other children to put up their hands if they thought of the same answer. If anyone had a different answer, he could ask them to say what it was.

Ideas for the classroom

It is very easy to make exercises in self-awareness and empathy part of your everyday teaching, even if you are not teaching about HIV and AIDS. These awareness exercises also encourage concentration in class.

1 Nurturing self awareness

At the beginning of your lessons, ask the children to close their eyes and take a deep breath. Allow them to be quiet for a moment and become aware of their bodies and how they feel. Are they relaxed? Are they tense? After a few moments ask them to take another deep breath and open their eyes.

2 Nurturing empathy

When you teach your lessons, make a point of encouraging children to think about the feelings involved. Here are some examples of the kind of questions you could ask when you are teaching English, Social Studies or Science.

- How do you think it feels to make a discovery?
- How do you think it feels to try something for the first time?
- How do you think it feels to know there will be a war?

Helpful hint

Empathy and self-awareness are ongoing processes. We rely on them every time we communicate.

49 Nurturing behaviour change

Did you know?

It is always easier to teach young people how avoid HIV infection if they are not yet having sex. It is much harder to encourage young people who are sexually active to abstain or to delay sex. That is why sex education should start as soon as children come to school.

Many young people are afraid to change their behaviour because they think their friends will laugh at them. Others want to change, but have no idea what to do. When adults criticise their behaviour, most young people become angry even if they agree that what they are doing is dangerous or wrong. (See also Topic 22 pages 46–47 and Topic 30 pages 64–65.)

The right approach

Research into the impact of HIV education has shown that the content of lessons is important, but that information alone does not change behaviour or protect our children from HIV.

'Preaching' too much and too loudly sometimes has the opposite effect to that intended. Pupils get bored with the 'HIV problem' and do not relate it to their own lives. That is why it is important to avoid a flood of information. It is better to concentrate on a few really important facts, and spend time with the pupils exploring the implications of these facts for their own lives. This takes time and trust.

Preventing pupils from getting bored

There are two useful ways in which teachers can prevent pupils from getting bored with discussing HIV and AIDS issues. Firstly, they must make sure there is no meaningless repetition. Secondly, they can check that the lessons are relevant to the pupils' lives. It often helps if teachers from different subject areas talk to each other about their plans and experiences in teaching children about HIV and AIDS.

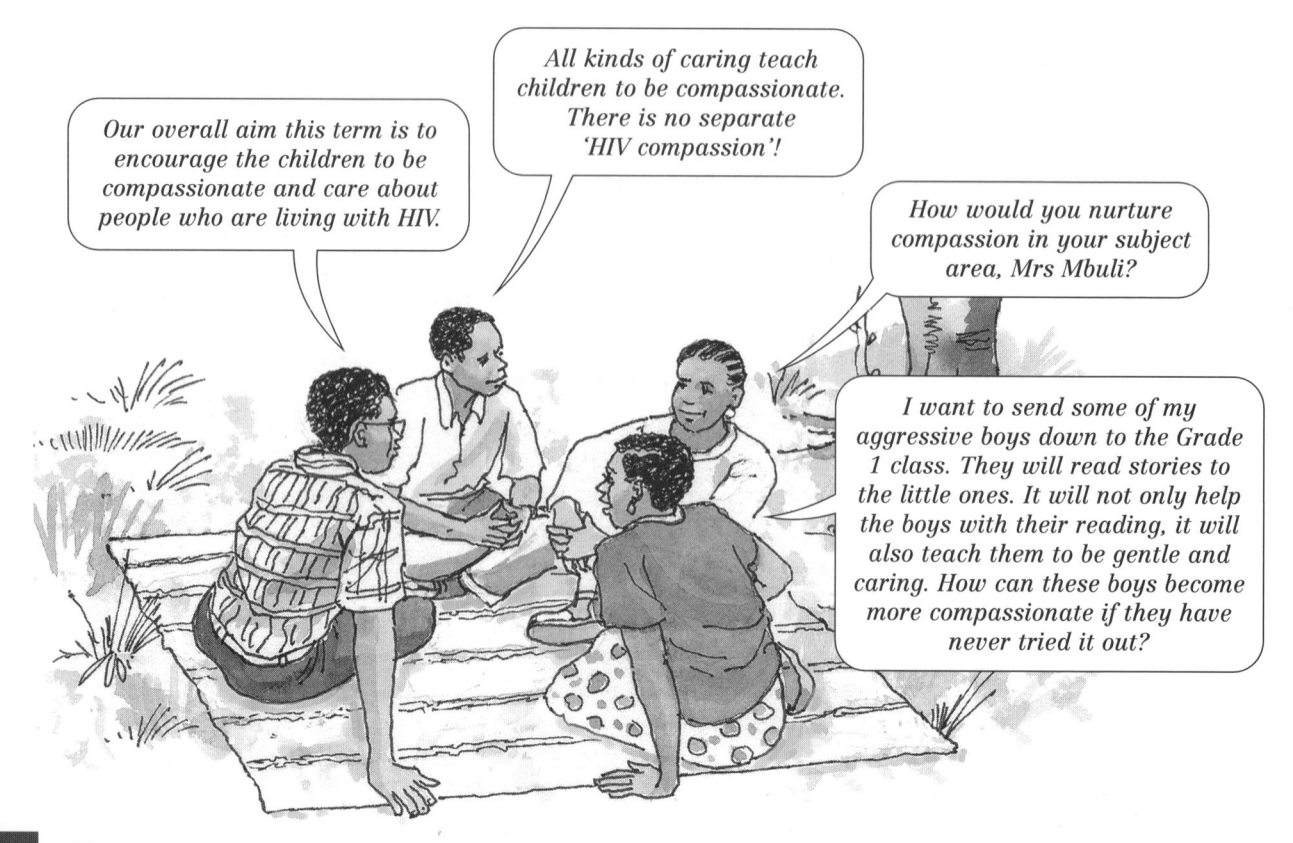

Our overall aim this term is to encourage the children to be compassionate and care about people who are living with HIV.

All kinds of caring teach children to be compassionate. There is no separate 'HIV compassion'!

How would you nurture compassion in your subject area, Mrs Mbuli?

I want to send some of my aggressive boys down to the Grade 1 class. They will read stories to the little ones. It will not only help the boys with their reading, it will also teach them to be gentle and caring. How can these boys become more compassionate if they have never tried it out?

Working together to encourage behaviour change

Teaching about HIV in all areas of the curriculum

Did you know?

The following help us to change:
- clear goals and expectations
- encouragement from friends
- noticing progress
- support from the family
- new friends who want the same as you.

The following make it hard to change:
- old habits
- unrealistic goals
- old friends laughing
- feeling lonely
- seeing no progress.

Case study

Mrs Mbuli is a teacher who has helped many pupils to change the way they behave. Her success comes from the fact that she does not talk about compassion, but rather gives her pupils an opportunity to experience it and to try it out. She does not expect the boys in her class to change without giving them a real opportunity to do so. She supports them to be caring rather than aggressive by:
- giving them a specific, but caring job to do
- taking them away from their peers, so they can try out 'being caring' without getting laughed at
- providing a familiar and safe environment (with a teacher in the school), which makes it easier to try something new.

Mrs Mbuli knows she is teaching the boys to be compassionate, but she does not have to tell them this. All she has to say to the boys is, 'We need your help in the Grade 1 class. Please go down to Ms Tete's class and she will tell you what to do.'

Activity Reflect on your own experience

Can your recall a time when you changed your behaviour? Revisit Topic 22, pages 46–47, which also discusses changes in behaviour.

Teaching about HIV and AIDS across the curriculum does not mean packing as much information as possible about HIV and AIDS into the lessons you teach. Rather, it means teachers begin to think of all subjects and all learning activities as opportunities to build the mental and moral capacity of learners for behaviour change.

Sound knowledge and caring values help young people to change their behaviour and choose an AIDS-free life.

Ideas for the classroom

Young people find it easier to abstain from sex or to delay having sex if they are taught less risky ways of spending time with their boyfriends and girlfriends. You can help them to delay having sex by:

- involving your class in school sports or drama activities
- organising walks and outings that allow young people to socialise together
- having a class party at the end of each term
- setting up dance, drama or other classes after school.

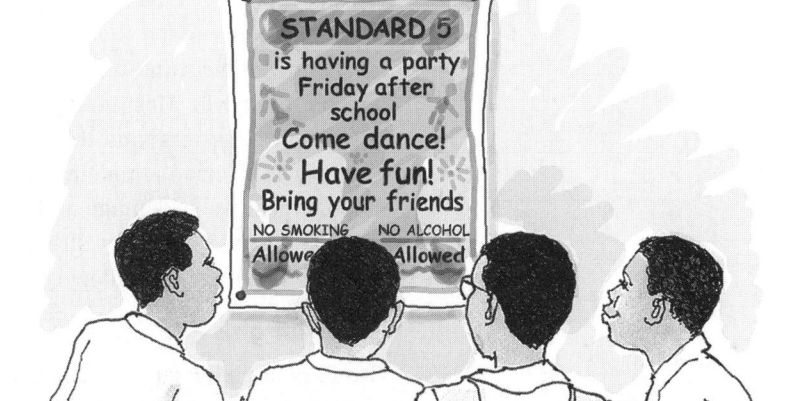

Helpful hints

- If you plan a social event in the evening, make sure the children are collected by their parents or other carers when the event ends.
- Some parents will be keen to help with social clubs and events. Involve them as much as possible.
- Always take some time to talk to the children about how you expect them to behave at these events. Clear expectations help with self-control.

50 Nurturing hope

The importance of hope

When Nelson Mandela became president of South Africa, he said these words:

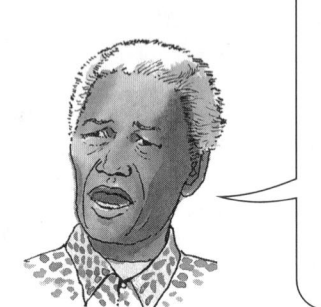

> Our deepest fear is not that we are inadequate.
> Our deepest fear is that we are powerful beyond measure.
> It is our light, not our darkness that most frightens us. ...
>
> As we let our light shine, we unconsciously give other people permission to do the same.
>
> As we are liberated from our fear,
> our presence automatically liberates others.
>
> *(Nelson Mandela, 1992)*

These words tell us a lot about hope.

Hope is more than a blind belief that things will turn out well. For Nelson Mandela, hope comes from knowing the right thing and choosing to do it, regardless of how things will turn out. People who have hope believe their lives are important and this gives them courage to do what is right. They also encourage others to imagine a better life for themselves.

Real hope changes people's behaviour and gives them a reason to live. Teachers who want to nurture the kind of hope Nelson Mandela speaks of will, therefore, take HIV and AIDS education seriously, regardless of what others think or say.

Feeling powerless and hopeless

Many young people find it hard to be hopeful, because they find it hard to love themselves. They find it hard to believe that their life is worthwhile and, as a result, they have no plans for the future. They simply stumble from one day to the next. Others wish they could be different, but feel too powerless to change.

This is especially true for girls. Many girls know, for example, that HIV is dangerous and that they should abstain from sex, but they also know of girls and women who have been forced to have sex against their will. Most girls grow up believing they have no choice about these matters, and this makes it hard for them to protect themselves. Nelson Mandela's words remind us that an attitude of hope, a positive self-image and good Life Skills are closely linked. They work together. They strengthen each other and all three are needed for behaviour change.

Hope for girls

There is hope for girls. It comes from:

- believing in their inborn right to live a healthy life

Activity What makes you feel hopeful about the future?

Can you think of an experience in your life where you became hopeful as soon as you had the courage to do the right thing?

Teaching about HIV in all areas of the curriculum

- having accurate knowledge of HIV and how it spreads
- imagining a better life for themselves
- being friends with other girls and boys who want to abstain from sex.

The need to praise children

Most parents and teachers want to protect children from problems and warn them to stay away from drugs, sex and violence that could destroy their lives.

They spend a lot of time and energy on trying to control what happens to the children they love. But do they spend enough time on building a positive self-image and teaching children how to make the right choices on their own? How much time do they spend telling children that they are wonderful or encouraging them to do their best? The warnings adults give children would be more effective if they also praised children for what they are doing right and celebrated their ability to succeed.

Activity   Two posters

Compare the two posters on this page. Which message do you prefer? Why? Which poster encourages a positive self-image. How?

Change the messages below so that they not only warn, but also encourage a positive self-image.

- Drugs can kill you!
- You could be infected. Get tested for HIV!

Helpful hints

- Encourage children to speak. They need to be active and participate in lessons so they can become confident about participating in life.
- Creativity and imagination take time. The first idea a child has is not always the best. Allow enough time for the children to try out more than one idea.

Ideas for the classroom

The following will nurture a sense of hope through creative thinking and problem solving, provided you are prepared to stand back and allow the children to speak.

1. Read or tell a short story.
2. Stop the story in the middle, at the point where there is a problem or a crisis that has to be solved.
3. Ask the children in your class to finish the story on their own.
4. Talk to the children about the endings they have created. Whose ending is the most hopeful? Why?
5. If you wish, you can read the real ending of the story and see if it is as good as the endings the children made up.

Section 6 Teaching children affected by HIV and AIDS

51 HIV and AIDS and vulnerable children

Definition

Vulnerable children are those who do not have a lot of support and can easily be hurt.

Why vulnerable children need extra care

Most social problems make children more vulnerable to HIV infection. We have seen this elsewhere in this book – see especially Topic 7, pages 16–17, Topic 20, pages 42–43 and Topic 40, pages 86–87.

Poverty, for example, does not cause HIV, but the need for money often forces young children into relationships that put them directly at risk of getting HIV. There is also a greater chance that children who are abused or emotionally neglected will become infected with HIV.

Telling these children about HIV and AIDS is very important, but this alone will not be enough to keep them safe. Once they are in a sexual relationship, they have little power to insist on safer sex. Vulnerable children, therefore, need extra care and support from the local community, so their needs can be met in a way that does not put them at risk of getting HIV.

There are many vulnerable children in Africa. Here are some of the most common problems these children have to face:
- hunger
- lack of parental support
- poverty and unemployment
- violence in the home
- emotional neglect
- abuse
- loss or absence of a parent
- insecurity.

What can the school and community do?

The school community can do four important things to make children less vulnerable to HIV.

1. Encourage children to go to school for as long as possible.
2. Teach them about HIV and AIDS.
3. Create a child-friendly and caring environment at school.
4. Communicate with parents and caregivers about the physical and emotional needs of the child.

Activity *Identifying problems*

Look at the list of problems that make children vulnerable.
- Which of these affect children in your area?
- How do these problems affect the children's performance at school?
- Which problems become worse when children live in a family that is affected by HIV or AIDS?

Teaching children affected by HIV and AIDS

Activity *Identifying vulnerable children*

How do you identify vulnerable children who need extra care and support?

Use this list as a guide. Add any other ideas that you have found useful.

Children need care and support when:

- they fall behind in their schoolwork
- they no longer pay attention in class
- they come to school hungry
- they feel lonely and helpless
- they are grieving the death of someone they loved
- they become silent and refuse to talk
- they are teased and bullied by others
- they can't pay school fees
- they live without parents and care for younger siblings

....
....
....
....
....

Finding better solutions

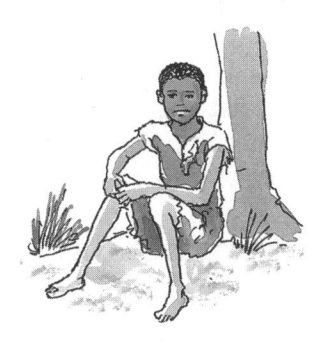

Problem: A child in need

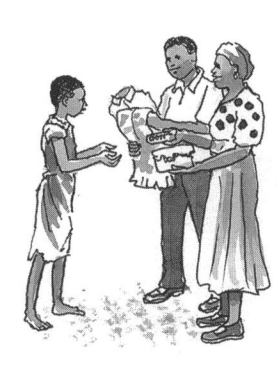

Solution: Help from relatives

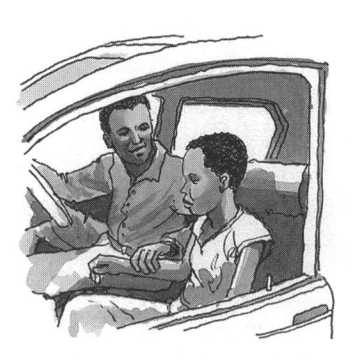

Problem: A man offers money to a girl in return for sex.

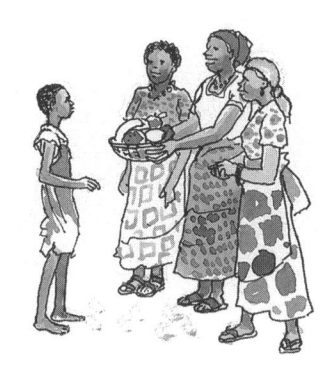

Solution: The community can help poor children so they do not need to put themselves in danger.

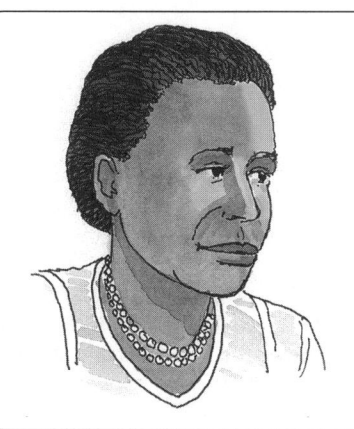

Case study

I am Mrs Sangoni, and I have been a principal for many years. Life has never been easy, but now since HIV came to our village things are worse. Most children are raised by grandmothers or come from single-parent homes. Now with the problem of AIDS, many children are left to somehow grow up on their own. Even if older sisters and brothers are responsible for their siblings they often lack parenting skills and have no support.

This causes social problems in the community and at our school. More and more children don't know how to behave and it is very difficult to teach them well. As a principal I have a responsibility to teach the children basic rules of social life, especially if they do not learn these rules at home.

Idea for the classroom

Do a vulnerability survey of your class. This will help you to know the children you are teaching and will make you more empathetic towards them. You can help to make children less vulnerable by making them feel loved or by appointing a 'helper' who will assist them to catch up the work if they have been absent for a long time.

52 Understanding vulnerable children

HIV and AIDS cause many problems at home or in the community. There are children who lose parents and care-givers. There are children who are running a household, and have little time for schoolwork. There is growing poverty in many communities, and illness among teachers and parents leaves children with little support.

How vulnerable children may behave

All of these factors have a strong influence on the classroom. They make it more difficult for children to learn.

Children are very vulnerable if they have social needs. They quickly feel unsettled and insecure. When teachers talk about HIV and AIDS in the classroom, some children become restless, wanting to disrupt the lesson that is causing them emotional pain. Others become quiet and refuse to participate at all, because they are afraid their friends will find out about the illness in their home. On the surface, these children seem naughty or lazy, but it is important for teachers to recognise that naughty behaviour can be a way of hiding difficult feelings and coping with social needs.

Social problems often affect the way children behave at school. Some children feel worried or lonely; others feel excluded. Many are afraid of being teased. There are children who become angry and fight a lot, and children who withdraw.

The chart on the next page shows some 'naughty' behaviours that tell you children are unhappy and might be affected by social problems outside of school.

Ideas for the classroom

Talk to children about their needs.

Ask the children to work in groups. Each group should make a list of things they feel they need so that they can do their best at school. Each group then reports their needs to the whole class.

Once the children have shared their ideas, talk about the needs they have presented. Are these needs met at present? How can you as a teacher help to meet these needs? How can the class work together to offer care and support for those in need?

End the lesson by asking each learner to complete the following sentences.

- My biggest need is ....
- I can help to meet this need by ....

Helpful hints

- Take time to observe the children in your care. You can do this when you are on playground duty, or when you are waiting for them to settle down at the beginning of class. Look at them as unique individuals. Look for their beauty and their dignity.
- Ask yourself, 'What does this child need?'

Teaching children affected by HIV and AIDS

Activity Looking at difficult behaviours

- Look at the behaviours in the table on this page.
- Underline the behaviours that are most common at your school.
- What does this tell you about the children's needs?

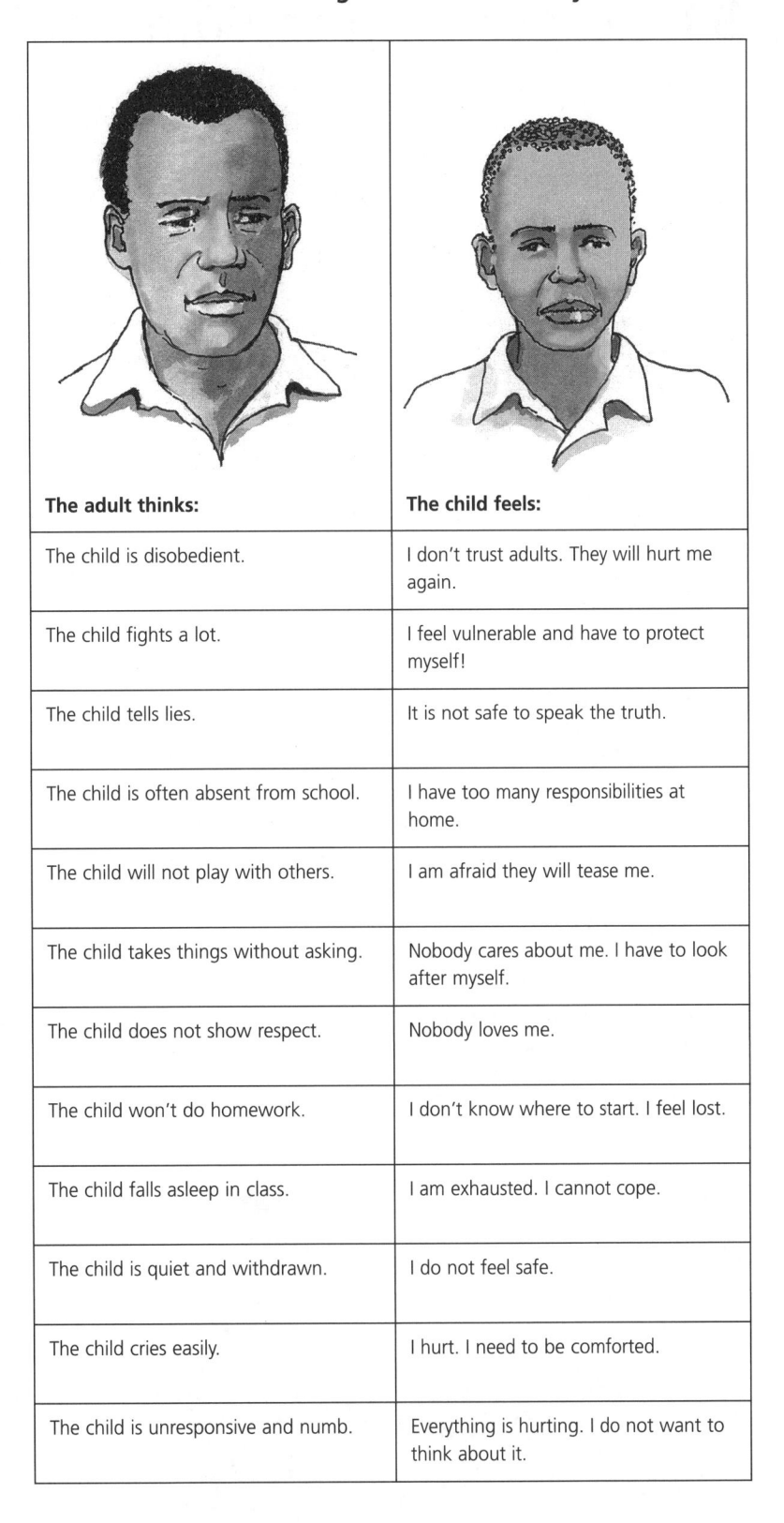

The adult thinks:	The child feels:
The child is disobedient.	I don't trust adults. They will hurt me again.
The child fights a lot.	I feel vulnerable and have to protect myself!
The child tells lies.	It is not safe to speak the truth.
The child is often absent from school.	I have too many responsibilities at home.
The child will not play with others.	I am afraid they will tease me.
The child takes things without asking.	Nobody cares about me. I have to look after myself.
The child does not show respect.	Nobody loves me.
The child won't do homework.	I don't know where to start. I feel lost.
The child falls asleep in class.	I am exhausted. I cannot cope.
The child is quiet and withdrawn.	I do not feel safe.
The child cries easily.	I hurt. I need to be comforted.
The child is unresponsive and numb.	Everything is hurting. I do not want to think about it.

53 Responding to vulnerable children

Definition

The **learning environment** is made up of three things:

1 the actual classroom and how it looks (physical)
2 the 'feeling' created in the class (emotional)
3 the way people relate (social).

Building up relationships

Through their day-to-day contact with their pupils, teachers are building the relationships that can support children in times of need. Children who experience a caring learning environment at school will have more confidence to cope with problems they face. This is especially important for children affected by HIV. Even if teachers are not able to change the suffering caused by the HIV epidemic, they can create a learning environment that will nurture the children along the way.

Comparing learning environments

A caring learning environment can build confidence and help children to succeed. Look at the two pictures on this page. The teacher on the left is impatient and threatening. She does not offer any support along the way. As a result, the child feels very vulnerable and is too afraid to learn.

The teacher on the right, however, is responding to the needs of the child. She notices that he is vulnerable, and so she thinks about the difficulties he might have. She decides not worry about the child's mistakes, but rather gives him practical help to overcome his problems. She encourages him to try. Her good methodology and her caring attitude make it possible for the child to become more confident and to do well at school.

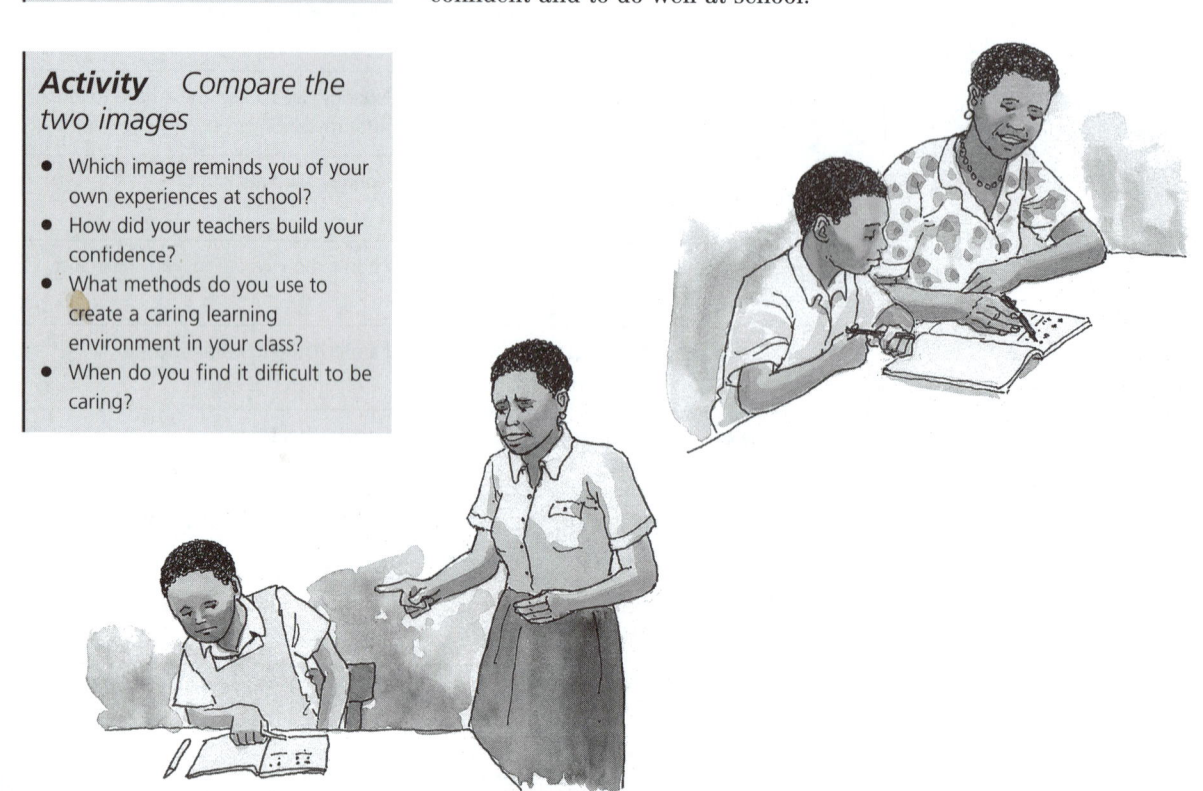

Create a child-friendly and safe school

- Have fair school rules.
- Know all the children by name.
- Be understanding.
- Praise the children as often as you can.
- Do not beat the children.
- Do not insult or verbally abuse children.
- Never touch inappropriately, kiss or have sex with a pupil.

Activity   Compare the two images

- Which image reminds you of your own experiences at school?
- How did your teachers build your confidence?
- What methods do you use to create a caring learning environment in your class?
- When do you find it difficult to be caring?

Teaching children affected by HIV and AIDS

The challenge of vulnerable children

It is emotionally and professionally challenging for teachers to respond to the needs of vulnerable children, especially as their numbers are increasing. Teachers need to talk to their colleagues about the challenges they face and how best to deal with them, sharing ideas. Some teachers worry about the level of discipline in their class. They think that if they show too much caring, they will look weak and lose their authority over the children. The case study is about Mr Jamba, a teacher in Tanzania, who is both strict and kind.

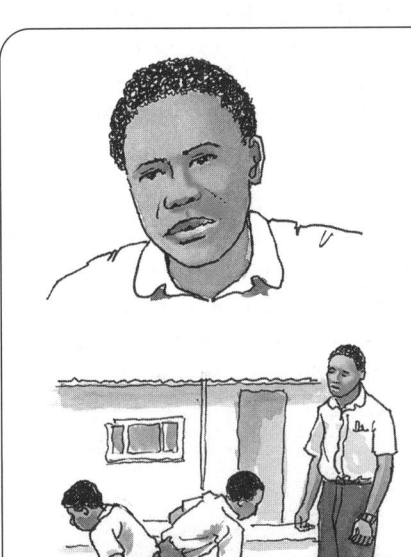

Case study

Mr Jamba is very strict, but he also cares for the children in his school. Here he talks about the secret of his success.

'The children know I am serious about learning.

I arrive on time for my lessons and I am always well-prepared. I also try to prepare my lessons in such a way that all children can participate, including the slow learners. I do not waste time in class and so the children have little chance to misbehave.

I have clear class rules, so all the children know exactly what I expect of them. They also have to be on time. I expect them to be polite. They must tell me if they could not do their work. I do believe that clear and consistent rules help children to succeed.

I believe it is important to set a good example and to deal with behaviour problems immediately. It is not good to let things grow. When I discipline my class I always tell the children what I find unacceptable and why it is breaking the rules. Then I try to think of a punishment that will help the children to improve. I may ask them to clean up the yard or stay behind to finish work.

My classes know I respect them and so I can expect to be respected in return.'

Ideas for classroom

Draw up clear rules to help children relate to each other in a caring and respectful way. Here are some examples of such rules. Notice that all these rules give positive messages about learning, and they also build self-confidence. They show the children that you trust them to do the right thing.

- Every child in this class is loved.
- We do not laugh or tease if somebody makes a mistake.
- We are proud of ourselves and will try our best.
- First we work, then we play.
- We talk about our feelings.
- When we are too angry to talk, we run up and down until we are ready. We can also ask a teacher to help us sort out a fight.

Allow the children to comment and add ideas to your list. By involving them in setting up the rules, you are encouraging them to keep them.

Helpful hints

Try to see mistakes and discipline problems as learning opportunities for both you and the child.

Always mention something good the child did, before you point out a mistake. This makes it easier to listen to the correction and many children will try again.

54 Supporting children with emotional needs

All children have emotional needs. All children need to feel secure and know that they are loved. They long for praise and their deep need for love and acceptance makes them vulnerable to other people, especially people they care about.

Taking children seriously

The best way of supporting children with emotional needs is to take their feelings seriously and to encourage them to express how they feel inside. A child who is able to talk about emotions will be able to cope better in times of stress or grief. Understanding emotions is, therefore, a very important life skill for children affected by HIV.

The first four years of schooling are a critical time in the emotional development of a child. It is the time during which their self-concept is being formed. This means primary school teachers have a lot of influence over the way children feel about themselves and about others. It is important to know that the way you deal with emotions in class will affect the children's emotional development and their self-esteem.

Activity *Reflect on your own upbringing*

- How did you learn about your emotions and how to handle them?
- How confident do you feel about supporting children in their emotional development?

(See also Topic 17, pages 36–37.)

Feelings

Children need help to learn the names of different feelings and what they mean. Discuss the positive feelings first and then the negative ones.

- What does love feel like?
- What is feeling happy like?
- What is feeling confident like?
- What does it feel like to be shy?
- What about fear?
- How do you know you are sad?
- What does anger feel like?

You can use stories and pictures from newspapers to help children notice different feelings and to talk about them.

How children react to crises

When families are in crisis, children quickly become aware that something is wrong. They can feel there is a problem, but they do not have enough information to work out what is going on. They realise that life is not always simple and not always safe. They need help with the insecurity they feel.

Unfortunately many families do not talk to the younger children about the problems they have. They have no time and energy to pay attention to the children's emotional needs. As a result, the children often feel excluded and alone. They feel unloved and, because their basic emotional needs are not met, they become unhappy and develop low self-esteem.

Teaching children affected by HIV and AIDS

Teachers may not be social workers or trained counsellors, but they can learn to listen well. Here are some guidelines you can use to improve the way you communicate with children with emotional needs.

Activity *Evaluate your own listening skills*

What are you good at? Where can you improve?

Steps to improving communication

Step 1: A helpful environment

Create a quiet space, where there are no distractions.
Make sure the child knows you have time.

Step 2: An accepting posture

Show with your posture that you are interested in what the child is saying. Look at the child. Lean forward to listen. Now and then you can nod, to show that you are listening.

Step 3: An open mind

Try not to make assumptions and listen with an open mind. Do not interrupt. Do not judge. Listen with an 'inner ear', paying attention to emotions rather than facts.

Step 4: Self-awareness

Notice what you are feeling while you are listening. Control your own emotions. Do not be afraid of silence.

Helpful hints

- If you are teaching children who are upset and sad, it is even more helpful than usual to set clear rules and limits. This helps them to experience a sense of security and predictability, while they are with you in class.
- Be kind and acknowledge their feelings. You do not have to solve the problem. Listening itself helps.

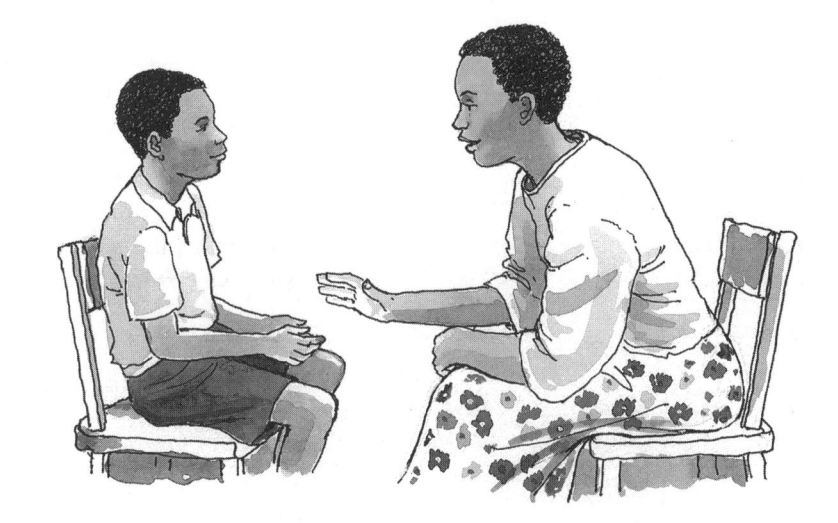

Remember

Children with high self-esteem feel good about themselves and take pride in what they do. They know what they are good at and find it easier to deal with peer pressure. High self-esteem helps young people to make good choices for their lives. It also helps them to take care of themselves and stay free of HIV.

Ideas for the classroom

Teach children to know and express different emotions by asking them to say 'Good morning' using different emotions, tone of voice and facial expressions. Tell them to, 'Say a "happy" good morning! Now say it in an angry way! Now say it as if you were afraid!' etc. Allow children to express their anger by tearing up old newspapers, or shouting loud in an empty room or hitting a ball as hard as they can. Emphasise that it is not OK to express your anger by hurting other people.

55 Discussing death with children

Definition

Emotional trauma is caused by intense emotional pain. The death of a person you love is a traumatic experience.

Activity An imaginary lesson

Imagine you have to teach a lesson about death to a primary school class. How would you answer these questions?

- What happens when people die?
- Why do people die?
- Why are we sad when people die?
- Can you stop people from dying?

Activity Imagine you are Marian

- How would you respond to Marian's problem? (See Case Study below.)
- Her adopted son is very angry. What other feelings could come up when he thinks about the fact that his parents died and left him behind alone?
- How could Marian respond to these feelings?

Approaching a discussion of death

There are many cultural reasons why adults find it difficult to talk to children about death.

Some people believe it is bad luck to mention death. Others feel children must be at least nine or ten years old before they are ready to talk about death.

In many cultures, children are not allowed to attend funerals and are protected from their parent's grief. This means many children in primary school are not prepared for the trauma of losing a parent or family member to AIDS.

How teachers can help with the trauma of death

Although the death of a person you love is always a traumatic experience, it is easier for children to respond to emotional trauma if they have been prepared for it. Teachers are not part of the immediate family, and so they can play an important role in helping children understand death and deal with pain and grief.

Children between six and twelve years have a concrete and practical understanding of death. They know that everyone has to die and that there are different causes of death. They also know that those who have passed on do not return. They are fascinated by details such as coffins, burial rituals, even decomposition and afterlife. They worry about death, because they do not want to be left behind alone.

Primary school children benefit from having accurate, factual information about death and about why people have died. They also find a lot of comfort in being able to talk about death. They need to tell their story and express their feelings, worries or questions.

Case study

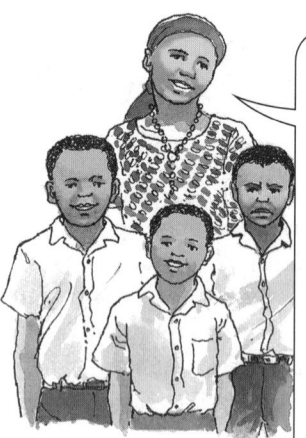

My name is Marian. I live in Uganda and work as a teacher in a primary school near Kampala. I am married and am raising three boys.

Not all of them are my own biological children. My middle son is my sister's child. He lost his parents to AIDS and I took him in when he was two. Now he is ten, and he is beginning to ask me a lot of questions about his mother and about how she died. I try to answer his questions, but it is difficult for me.

You see, his parents did not want everybody in the family to know that they were suffering from AIDS. So now I feel I have to respect their wishes and cannot tell the boy the truth. But he wants to know what happened and is beginning to blame me for the fact that his parents died.

The other day he was very angry with me and very rude. He said I poisoned his mother and that is why she died. It hurts me to hear this, because I cared for him when he had nobody else. What should I do?

Teaching children affected by HIV and AIDS

Ideas for the classroom

Read stories to children, in which somebody loses a loved one and has to grieve. Stories can help children to identify with others and to get to know their own feelings.

Use your Social Studies lessons to teach the children about the funeral rituals in your area. What symbols are used? What do they mean? What songs are sung? What clothes do people wear?

You can encourage children to understand their feelings about death through art, role-play or music.

For example, move the class outdoors where they have space to move. Let them stand in a big circle. Now give the children clear instructions like this:

- When somebody dies we feel sad. Slowly move around the circle, so we can see the sadness in your body. Move in a sad way.
- Some people get very angry. Move in an angry way.
- Move in a hurt way.
- Move in a lonely way, in a comforted way, in a panicky way – and so on.

Use a drum or a shaker to create a rhythm so all the children move at the same time.

Change the rhythm of the drum to go with the emotions. A sad rhythm is slow. An angry rhythm is fast.

Helpful hints

- Be honest with the children.
- There are many questions about death that do not really have an answer. It is good for children to understand this from an early age.

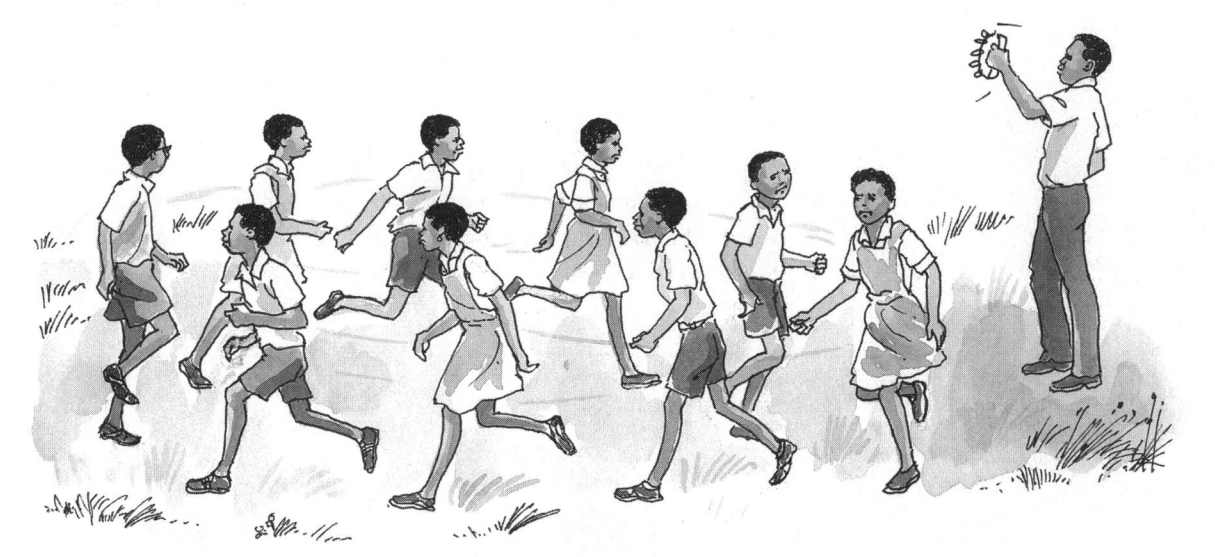

56 Supporting children in times of grief

When children are orphaned by AIDS

In many countries, there is still a lot of fear, superstition, guilt and rejection surrounding AIDS. As a result, people are scared to test for HIV. If they know they are infected, they are careful about whom to tell.

This means that many children who are orphaned as a result of the HIV epidemic might not know that their parents died of AIDS. Others might notice the symptoms, but feel too shy or afraid to ask their family about it. Some children might even be given wrong information about the way their parents died.

The negative effects of emotional trauma

When children are surrounded by secrecy and uncertainty, they find it especially hard to cope with emotional pain. A negative response to emotional trauma can affect them for many years to come. They can grow up believing they have no control over their lives or that they are helpless and weak.

Here are some of the negative responses that make it hard for children to accept the death of a person they love:

- Children believe it is their fault their parents died.
- Children become fearful and find it hard to trust others.
- Children develop angry feelings and find it difficult to ask for help.
- Children begin to worry, feel exhausted and depressed.

(See also Topic 10, pages 22–23; Topic 17, pages 36–37; and Topics 51 and 52, pages 108–111.)

When a family is affected by HIV or AIDS, children watch their parents or siblings becoming weaker and weaker. They start to worry about the future and often are afraid of having to survive on their own. They worry about questions such as:

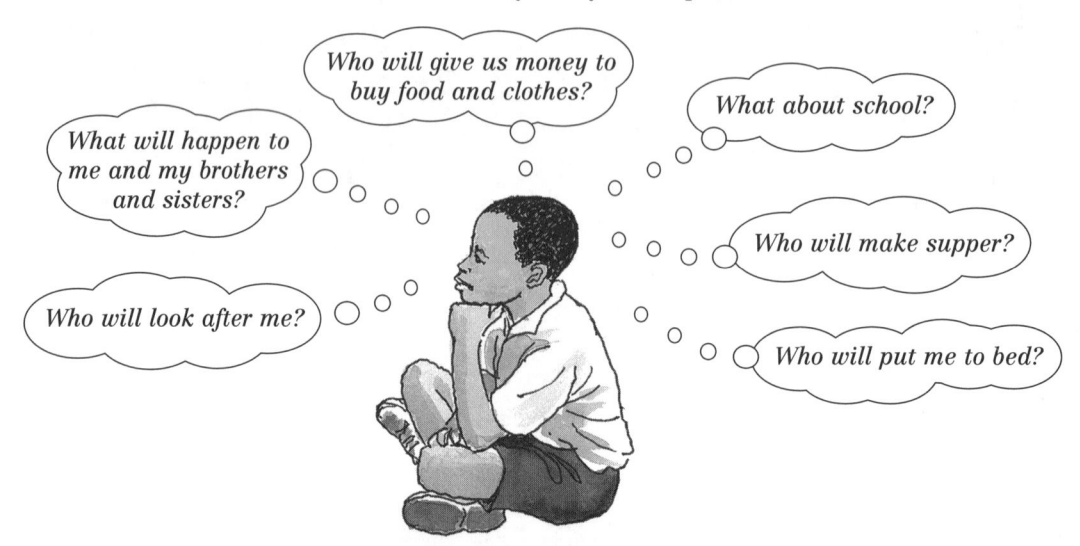

Who will give us money to buy food and clothes?

What about school?

What will happen to me and my brothers and sisters?

Who will make supper?

Who will look after me?

Who will put me to bed?

Teaching children affected by HIV and AIDS

Breaking with tradition

Traditionally, people do not talk openly about death to their children. In the face of AIDS, however, more and more parents in Africa are looking for ways to prepare their children for a time when they might have to cope without parental guidance and support. They believe that children need to know who will care for them after the mother or father dies, and they should be given detailed information about themselves and their families, so the death of a parent does not lead to a loss of identity for the child. Teachers can also play an important role in supporting children in times of grief.

> *Helpful hint*
>
> When children are grieving, teachers share the burden of their grief. This can be exhausting. Allow yourself to cry for the children in your care.

> *Activity* *Encouraging strong self-concepts*
>
> The list below contains a variety of areas in which teachers can encourage children to develop a strong self-concept and help them to cope with grief.
>
> - Provide a secure and happy learning environment at school.
> - Help them understand what HIV is, and how it affects people's lives.
> - Encourage them to be proud of their history and cultures, and always to try to find out more.
> - Plan differentiated lessons so all children can experience success. (See Topic 57, pages 120–121.)
> - Nurture positive and healthy relationships with the children in your class.
> - Appreciate the children's efforts and use lots of praise.
> - Act as a role-model for the children.
> - Encourage them to talk about their experiences and listen with a caring attitude.
>
> Are there any other ideas you would like to add? Plan a lesson, keeping in mind

Ideas for the classroom

Encourage children to know the history of their family. Ask them to find out where their grandparents came from and what it was like when their parents were young. How did their parents meet? Where did they live? What did they like to do?

Encourage children to draw or write about family celebrations or special family events.

Together with the parents or caregivers, draw up an 'I am not alone' card, recording their ID number, their home address, the names of their closest family and the names of people they should turn to in times of need. If possible, include a photo of the child with people they love.

Show compassion for children who are grieving and encourage other children in class to make cards or write messages of support.

Do a project on family memories, encouraging children to write about the people they love and miss. (See also Topic 46, pages 98–99.)

57 Teaching large classes

> **Definition**
>
> **Differentiated teaching** means that the whole class is working on the same content, but the teacher has prepared different tasks for different levels of ability.

Problems for children and their teachers

Children's problems

Children affected by HIV often find it hard to pay attention to their work. This is especially true for children who are traumatised or who are struggling with the impact of HIV on their family and their lives. When children find life difficult, they work more slowly than others. They also need extra encouragement and support. Often they do not finish or miss out on whole sections of their work.

Teachers' problems

A large class is a difficult environment in which a teacher may have to support children affected by HIV. There is not enough time to help learners catch up on the work they have missed. Many teachers feel frustrated, because the large class sizes make it difficult for them to do a good job. They know they are not reaching all the children and so they worry about the quality of their work.

> *Activity* Get to know the children in your class
> - How do you remember the names of all the children in your class?
> - How many slow learners are in your class?
> - How do you help them to keep up with the rest of the class?

Ideas for the classroom

Differentiated lessons

While some children fall behind, others are quick to finish their work. They get bored and restless while they wait for the rest of the class to catch up. A teacher who is teaching large classes needs some strategies to make sure all children are meaningfully busy all the time.

One way of responding to different learning needs of a large class is to teach a differentiated lesson. This means the teacher plans the lesson in such a way that slow learners are doing a task that is a little different, so they can finish in time. Teachers who differentiate their lessons believe that 'less is more'. It is better for a child to do less work and to do it well, than to try a lot of work that never gets finished. All children start their work at the same time and all finish at the same time. The task for the children who struggle has to be short enough, so they can do it in the given time.

> *Did you know?*
>
> Differentiated teaching is not only for children affected by HIV. It can help all children succeed.

Teaching children affected by HIV and AIDS

Activity A differentiated lesson plan

Look at this differentiated lesson plan for a 30 minute lesson. It is based on Topics 20 and 21. (See pages 42–45.)
Which activity is for learners who struggle to finish?
How could you use this kind of planning in your class?

Class: 1

Lesson: My body is my own and must be respected

Lesson introduction: All children sing a song, naming their body parts, while teacher points to part of the body. (5 minutes)

Demonstration of task: Teacher points to drawing of body on the board. Introduces the idea of 'private' body parts and tells children not to let anybody else play with their private body parts. (5 minutes)

	Group 1	Group 2	Group 3
10 minutes	Pupils should come to the desk and work with the teacher to identify private body parts, and say what 'private' means. **Assessment:** The teacher checks understanding while working with group.	The children work in a group, copying a drawing of the body from the board. They colour in the body sections that are private.	The children work in a group, each child making a drawing of their own body, colouring in the private sections, writing their name underneath.
5 minutes	The children work in a group, copying a drawing of the body from the board.	**Assessment:** The teacher checks drawings of this group and checks that they understand what 'private' means.	The children then look at each other's pictures and try to think of a 'message sentence' to say that children's bodies must be respected, for example, 'My body is my own.'
5 minutes	The group continues to colour picture. This gives them enough time to finish the task.	The group sits down and works on their own 'message sentence' to say that children's bodies must be respected, for example, 'My body is my own.'	**Assessment:** The teacher checks the work of the group and writes the message on the board for all to see.

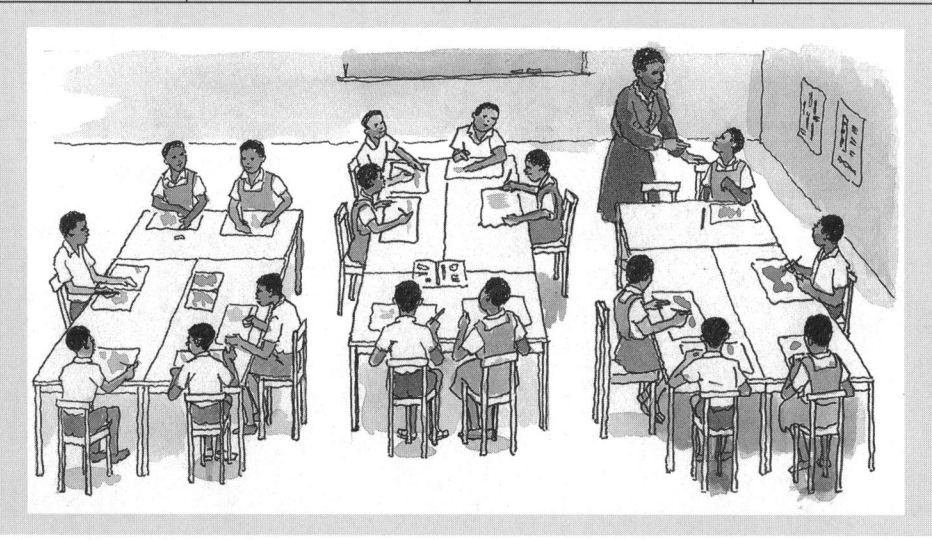

58 Supporting children who are absent from school

When children fall behind

When children are affected by HIV or AIDS they often stop coming to school. This is a problem for teachers because the children miss out on classes and fall behind in their work.

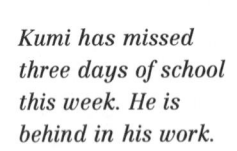

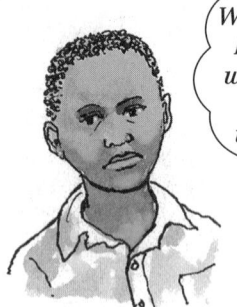

Kumi has missed three days of school this week. He is behind in his work.

Will the teacher ask Kumi to catch up with everything, or only the really important tasks?

How can the teacher help Kumi cope with the lesson, despite his 'gaps'?

What can a teacher do to break this negative cycle?

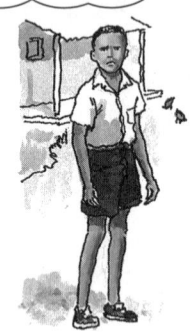

He struggles with his lessons, because he missed so much work. He is slow. He falls behind. He has no time to do the extra work he needs to do.

Who could help Kumi?

How can the teacher motivate Kumi to keep up?

Kumi gives up. He stops coming to school.

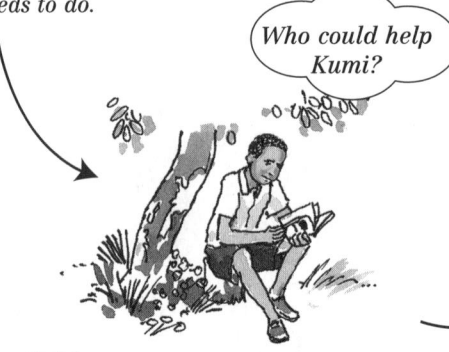

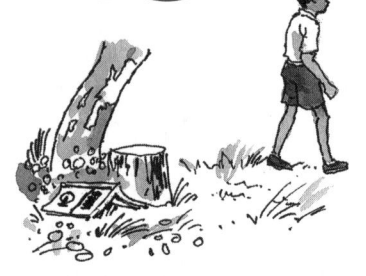

He tries to catch up with the work at home. He is not sure what to do. He tries, but has no help.

He does not finish his work. He is demotivated. He stops trying.

Activity   Talk about Kumi's story

What kind of help does Kumi need?

What can a teacher do to help Kumi succeed?

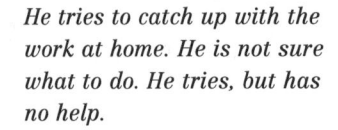

Teaching children affected by HIV and AIDS

> *Help children find their way back into school*
>
> When children drop out of school:
> - they are more vulnerable to HIV infection
> - they learn less about preventing the spread of HIV and AIDS
> - they have little support to develop safe behaviours.

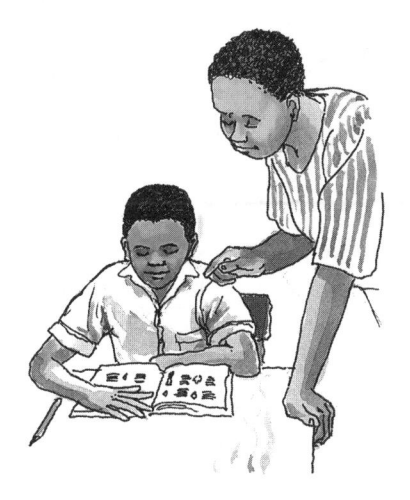

Ideas for the classroom

Some teachers support children who have been absent by offering extra lessons after school. This helps the children to catch up what they have missed. The extra lessons are also an opportunity for slow learners to get some extra help.

Many teachers appoint a 'helper' from the class to make sure the absent children catch up on the work. Often the helper is a very good and organised student who can explain the work. It also helps if children can copy the missing lessons from the books of children who are doing well at school.

Some schools are setting up 'homework clubs' among children who live in the same area. The children in the homework club always do their homework together, so they can help each other, even if one of them misses a day at school. Each homework group has a leader and the leader reports to the teacher the next day. The teacher can use the homework clubs to motivate and reward students to keep up with their work.

Some of the younger children find it helpful if the teacher puts up a homework chart in class. The homework chart is like a weekly timetable and shows what work has to be done each day of the week. The homework chart is also a help for teachers. When a child has been absent, the teacher can take one look at the week's work and choose only one or two really important tasks for the child to catch up.

Helpful hint

Don't worry if children do not catch up all the work. Think about the most important lessons they have missed, and make sure they catch them up. It is more important that they fit in with the lessons you are busy with at present. This keeps them motivated and helps them to keep pace when they return.

	Reading	Writing	Working with numbers	Subject:	Subject:	Project:
Monday						
Tuesday						
Wednesday						
Thursday						
Friday						

59 Creating caring classrooms for children with AIDS

Helpful hints

As we recall all the things we have talked about in this book, we know that it is most important that children with HIV or AIDS be included in all school activities as long as they are able. As teachers, we should be sure not to support the stigmatising of these children, or any person with HIV or AIDS. We may have to lead by example. With your fellow teachers, talk about ways that you can change negative attitudes in your school and community, if they exist.

Extra care and support

When children are beginning to show the first signs of AIDS, they need a lot of extra care and support at school. This can take many different forms.

Sometimes it is an *attitude*, expressed through public prayers, or in the accepting way teachers talk about HIV and AIDS.

Sometimes care and support is a charitable, *practical* response. This could include setting up a little rest area in the school or helping children with AIDS to keep up with their schoolwork.

In most cases children experience care and support as a *relationship*, lived out in the way teachers listen to their needs, the way they show compassion and they protect those who are vulnerable because of AIDS.

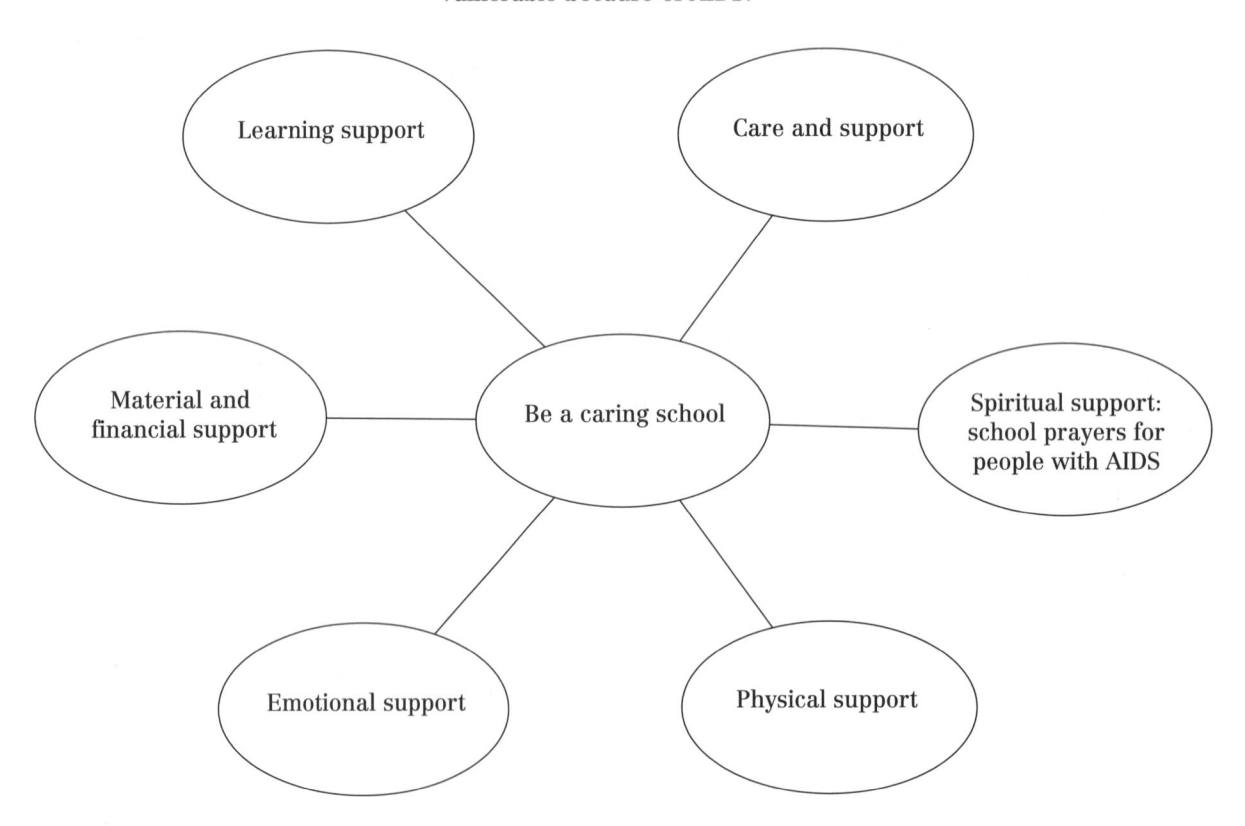

Mind map — Be a caring school:
- Learning support
- Care and support
- Material and financial support
- Spiritual support: school prayers for people with AIDS
- Emotional support
- Physical support

Activity Discuss the mind map

Copy the mind map and discuss it with your colleagues at school or with fellow students. What can schools do to provide a caring school environment for children with AIDS? Write your responses under the relevant headings of the mind map. For example, if you think schools can say prayers for people with AIDS, write that activity under the heading 'spiritual support'.

Teaching children affected by HIV and AIDS

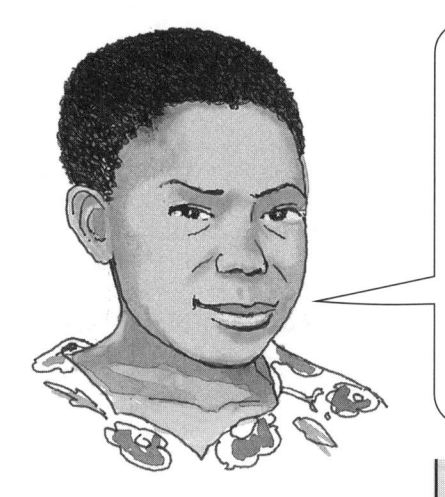

When you teach children who have AIDS, you will need to make some special arrangements to help them cope at school. For example, children may feel unwell during school-time and need to have access to a clean and quiet sick bay where they can lie down. When they are young, they need to have help with taking medication. Children with HIV often miss classes and tests and so I had to develop a flexible and creative approach to schoolwork.

Children with AIDS need to be protected from infection. This means that they need an environment that is hygienic: access to safe drinking water, hygienic food preparation, clean toilets and access to water so they can wash hands. They also need good, balanced nutrition. But, above all, they need to feel safe and loved.

Activity A checklist

Use this checklist to see whether your school is providing a safe and healthy environment for children with AIDS.

- Everybody at the school has access to clean water to wash their hands.
- We have enough toilets (pit-latrines or flush toilets).
- All our toilets are cleaned and fixed regularly.
- Sanitary pads are disposed of safely.
- Our classrooms are well ventilated.
- We always use universal precautions when dealing with blood or other body fluids. (See Topic 3, pages 8–9.)
- Our children eat at least one balanced meal a day.
- All food is prepared under clean and hygienic circumstances.
- We have a clean and private sick-bay.
- We treat medical information confidentially.
- We have made contact with our local clinic for support.

Activity Discussion points

- What worries you about teaching children with AIDS?
- What would worry other members of the school community?

Helpful hints

You do not have to provide all the care and support on your own. Rather, strengthen the existing support structures within the school, with the local clinic and with the family of the child.

Confronting social stigma

When teachers try to have caring relationships with children affected by AIDS, they are quickly confronted with the social stigma attached to the disease. They have to respond to prejudice, fear and hate. Many teachers try to break down prejudice by teaching children empathy and compassion for their classmates and other children in the school. (See Topic 15, pages 32–33.)

Ideas for the classroom

If you notice that some of your pupils are showing signs of AIDS, take time to talk to them, asking them how they are feeling and what kind of support they would like from the school.

You can also teach some general lessons on the different stages of AIDS. This will help everybody to know what to expect. For more information, see Section 1, pages 2–25.)

Communicate with the family so you know what they would like you to do when their children are feeling ill at school.

60 The value of home visits

How a teacher can help

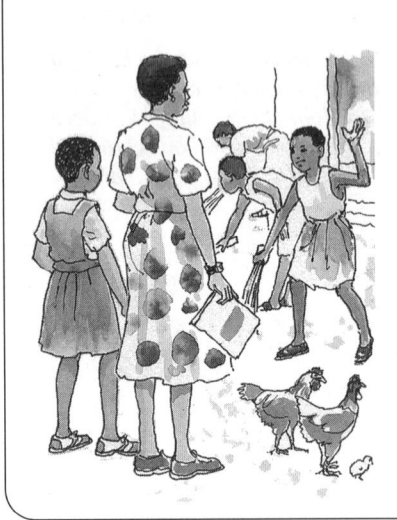

Case study

It is Miss Thobeka's first year as a senior primary teacher and she has not been in the village for long. She likes teaching, but her new class is so big that she still does not know all the children by name. On Wednesday, Sara came to her after school and said that she is worried because her best friend had not been in school all week. Miss Thobeka felt bad, because she had not noticed the missing girl.

'Do you know where your friend lives?' she asked.
'Yes,' said Sara.
'Shall we go and visit her?'

Together, Miss Thobeka and Sara set out to find the missing friend. When they got to her home, Jeneba was sweeping the yard with her three younger sisters. It didn't take Miss Thobeka long to find out that the house was stripped of all belongings and the children were left without food.

'My mother borrowed a lot of money to buy medicines,' Jeneba said, looking ashamed. 'Now that she has passed away, we are left alone. They came and took our things, because we owed them.'

Activity 1 Finish the story

- What do you think happened next?
- What is Miss Thobeka's responsibility in this situation?

Jeneba's story shows how important a home visit can be for children affected by HIV or AIDS. Although Miss Thobeka cannot provide all the care and support Jeneba needs, there are several things Miss Thobeka could do.

- **Immediate response**

She can show caring and compassion by listening to Jeneba's story. She can give Jeneba some food for the evening meal. She can ask Jeneba to come back to school the next day.

- **Short-term response**

She can talk to Jeneba at school and encourage her to catch up her work.

She can visit Sara's family and talk about ways in which friends and neighbours can help the children. She can contact a social worker, a priest or an NGO working with HIV/AIDS issues and tell them about Jeneba's need.

Activity 2 Considering your own response

- How would you respond to Jeneba's case?
- Who are the key partners in your community who can help care for children affected by HIV and AIDS?

- **Long term-response**

She can speak to the principal about Jeneba's school fees. She can encourage the school committee to find out how many other children like Jeneba drop out of school.

She can have a meeting to talk about the school's responsibility for children like Jeneba, who are destitute because of AIDS.

Teaching children affected by HIV and AIDS

Helpful hint

Home visits can start at your home. As a teacher you are part of a local community. Do you know the people around you? Where do their children go to school?

The ripple effect

It is difficult for schools to plan a long-term response to the needs of children affected by HIV and AIDS. Many families hide their problems and their need. That is why home visits are valuable. They help to connect the school with the families they serve. Every caring response during a home visit will have a ripple effect that can change the whole community. Here is the ripple effect that Sara's love for her friend had on her school:

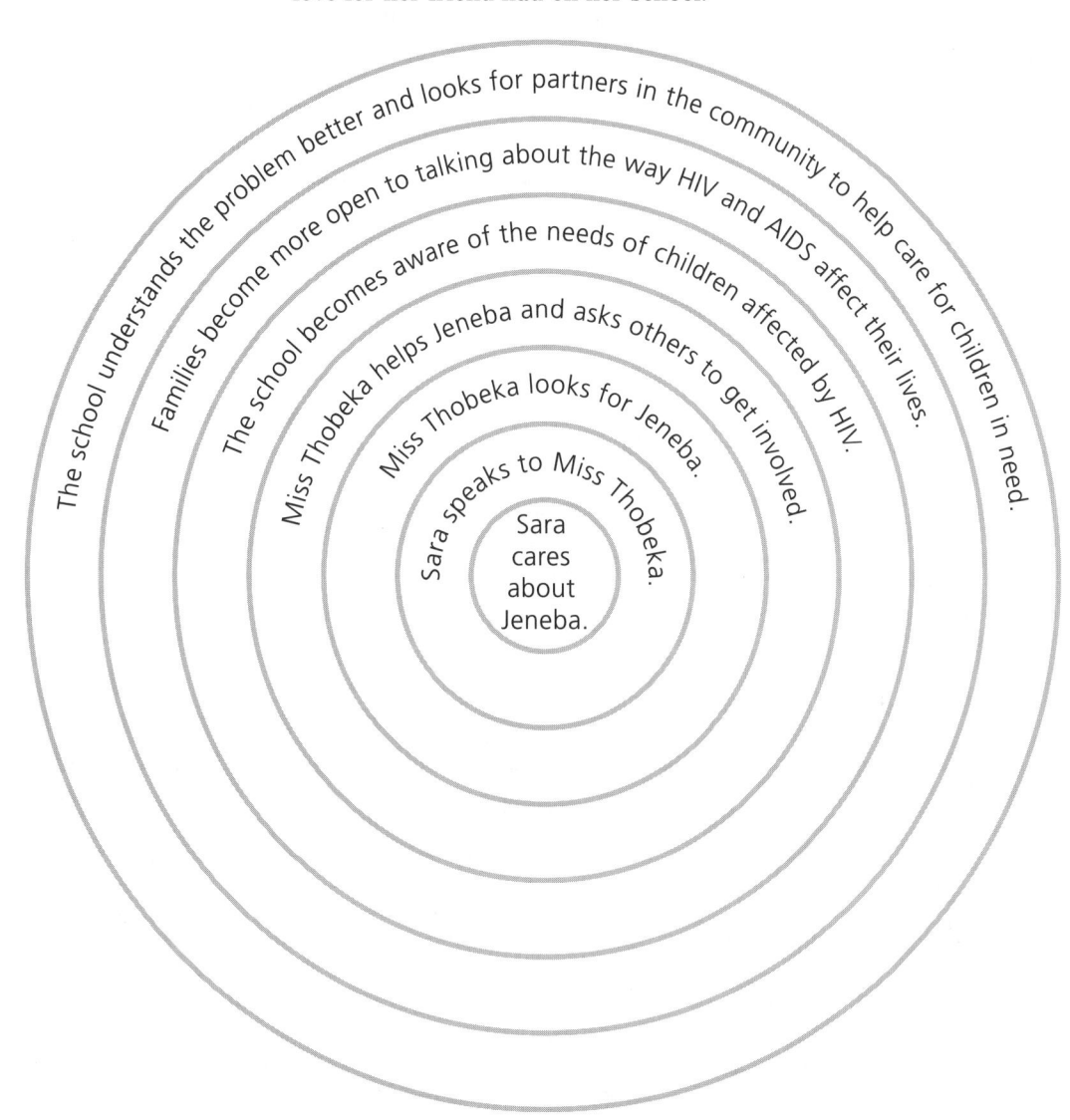

- Sara cares about Jeneba.
- Sara speaks to Miss Thobeka.
- Miss Thobeka looks for Jeneba.
- Miss Thobeka helps Jeneba and asks others to get involved.
- The school becomes aware of the needs of children affected by HIV.
- Families become more open to talking about the way HIV and AIDS affect their lives.
- The school understands the problem better and looks for partners in the community to help care for children in need.

Activity Reflect on your personal experience

Can you think of any situation where the simple, but caring, response of one person had a ripple effect through the whole community? What happened?

61 Who cares for the carers?

Definition

Having **emotional health** means feeling good about yourself and having the inner strength to cope with problems that come your way.

Looking after traumatised children

Teaching can be very exhausting, especially when you teach children who are traumatised, grieving or struggling to learn.

When teachers try to provide a caring learning environment for these children, they often end up acting as social workers and pastoral counsellors, parents and health workers in a community where many families are in need.

That is why we need to ask, 'Who cares for the carers?' How can teachers look after their own emotional health? Emotional health involves a variety of attitudes, habits and skills. It means loving and accepting yourself, feeling confident about your abilities, coping with stress and sadness and the general ups and downs.

Basic Life Skills

Basic Life Skills are the key to good emotional health. This is as true for teachers as everyone else. Some of the most important life skills for teachers include:

- maintaining high self-esteem
- maintaining self-confidence
- being able to cope with stress
- being able to cope with sadness
- developing self-awareness
- developing empathy
- knowing how to solve problems
- knowing how to communicate and negotiate
- developing assertiveness.

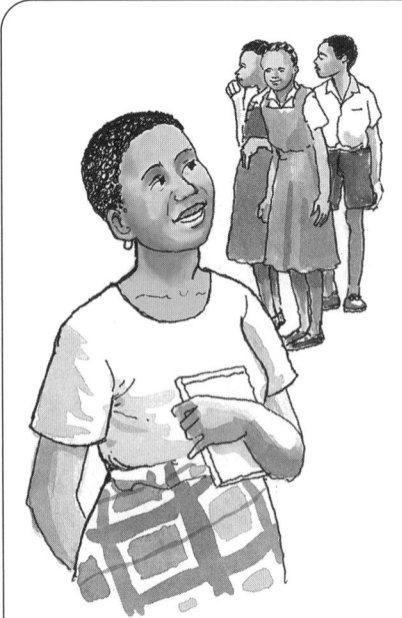

Case study 1

Mary Sekoto is an experienced teacher and has been at her school for many years. Although she has little formal training, she is confident in her work. She knows she has helped many children to become literate and does not get too worried when things don't turn out the way she had planned. She thinks of herself as a life-long learner and is not shy to ask for help when she is not sure what to do.

Sometimes she gets very tired and down-hearted because, since the HIV epidemic started in her community, children have more problems than before. When she feels down-hearted she talks to other teachers about her feelings. They remind her that she is a caring and dedicated teacher and deserves to take a rest when she is tired.

Her work makes an important difference in her school, even if she cannot solve all the problems the children face.

Teaching children affected by HIV and AIDS

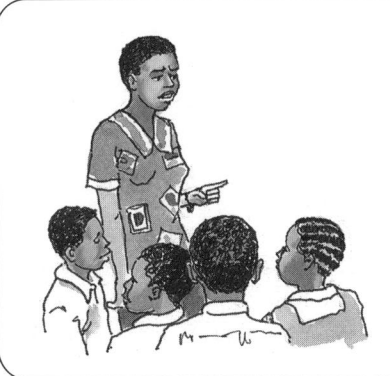

Case study 2

Grace Lulama finds it much harder to cope with the problems and disruptions caused by HIV. She feels demotivated, and often blames the children when they are absent from school.

With all the problems in the community, the children struggle to learn. Now the results of Mrs Lulama's classes are lower than before. She feels bad about this and worries what other people will say. She is angry that the problems slow down her teaching and now she can no longer finish all the work in time.

She feels dissatisfied and stressed a lot of the time, wishing the problems would simply go away.

Activity   A comparison

Compare Mrs Sekoto's and Mrs Lulama's responses to problems.

- Why is Mrs Lulama so worried?
- What helps Mrs Sekoto to stay positive and caring in the face of all the problems she faces in her work?

Mrs Lulama's story shows that the way you think about your job is greatly influenced by how other people judge the work you do. In societies where the teaching is losing status and credibility, many teachers feel under-valued and this affects their self-esteem. Mrs Sekoto's story reminds us that teachers can learn to protect themselves against these undermining feelings and actively build their confidence and self-esteem.

Here are some more ideas:

- Do not compare yourself with others. Set your own goals that are right for your situation, and be proud if you achieve them.
- Think about the kind of person you are, and list your best qualities.
- Think of your special talents, and make a list of the things you do well.
- Notice when you blame others for your problems. Blaming is often a sign that you need to take better care of yourself.
- Be realistic. Set achievable goals and celebrate your real achievements.
- Believe in yourself and be glad that you can grow and change.
- Spend time with people who care about you and make you feel good about yourself.

Activity   Your own responses

How do you respond when you feel exhausted?
How valued do you feel as a teacher in your community?
What abilities do you have that other people admire?
Make a list of your skills and competencies that help you succeed as a teacher.

When teachers get too exhausted, they can become depressed. They feel empty and hopeless when they think about their work. Often they also feel overwhelmed by all the problems they see. Here are some symptoms of depression:

- feeling sad or dull most of the time
- feeling without energy
- having difficulty sleeping or sleeping too much
- having muddled thoughts
- having regular headaches and stomach problems
- feeling unable to enjoy activities the way you used to in the past
- not wanting to see friends
- changing eating and drinking habits (especially an increase in sweets, alcohol) to try and ignore problems.

Answers to quiz questions throughout book

Answers

Topic 4: Activity
Evaluation answers
1. HIV is the infection that causes AIDS. Someone can have HIV and show no symptoms at all, but they are able to infect other people. AIDS is the illness caused by HIV, when the body's immune system can no longer fight infections.
2. Part 1 shows the window period – the virus has attached itself to the CD4 cells, but no reaction has started yet.
3. T-cells are an important part of the immune system, which fights off infections.

Topic 12: quiz answers
1F, 2F, 3F, 4F, 5T (so that she or he does not catch any illnesses), 6F.

Topic 15: the true reasons how the people got infected with HIV:
- David was infected with HIV when he helped someone at an accident.
- Hanna was infected when she decided to have sex with her neighbour for food.
- Beryl was infected when she was raped by a teacher while she was still at school.
- John was infected when he had unprotected sex with a woman from his church.

Now go back and see whether your sympathy for these people has changed.

Topic 38: quiz answers
1. False, there is no position that can prevent pregnancy. If the sperm goes inside the woman's vagina she can get pregnant. There is also no position that will keep you safe from HIV and AIDS.
2. False, there is some sperm in the liquid a man releases before he ejaculates.
3. False, it can happen that a woman gets pregnant even when menstruating. It is also especially dangerous to have unprotected sex during menstruation because the menstrual blood can contain or transmit HIV.
4. False, there are about 500 million sperm cells in a teaspoonful of sperm. It is impossible to wash all of these away.
5. False, boys at the age of 12 can already produce sperm.
6. False, it does not matter if a girl or woman is good or bad. If she has sex without using contraceptives, she can get pregnant.

Answers to quiz questions throughout book

7 False, there is a pill that can stop pregnancy, but only a condom can stop a man both from making a woman pregnant and from getting infected with HIV.

8 False, if sperm reaches an egg a girl or woman can get pregnant even the first time she had sex.

Topic 43: quiz answers

1 HIV is a virus.
2 HIV destroys the immune system of the body.
3 If the immune system of the body is not working properly, the body cannot fight off germs and diseases. This means that a person with HIV will easily get sick and even small infections can be very dangerous.
4 Through sex, from mother to child during pregnancy, birth and breastfeeding, through blood transfusion or sharing needles, razors etc. without sterilising them.
5 Abstain from sex, delay sex until you are older, take an HIV test before starting a sexual relationship, use condoms, be faithful for life with one faithful, tested partner, take care when there is a risk of coming into contact with another person's blood.

Teaching about HIV and AIDS

Picture story: A dangerous situation

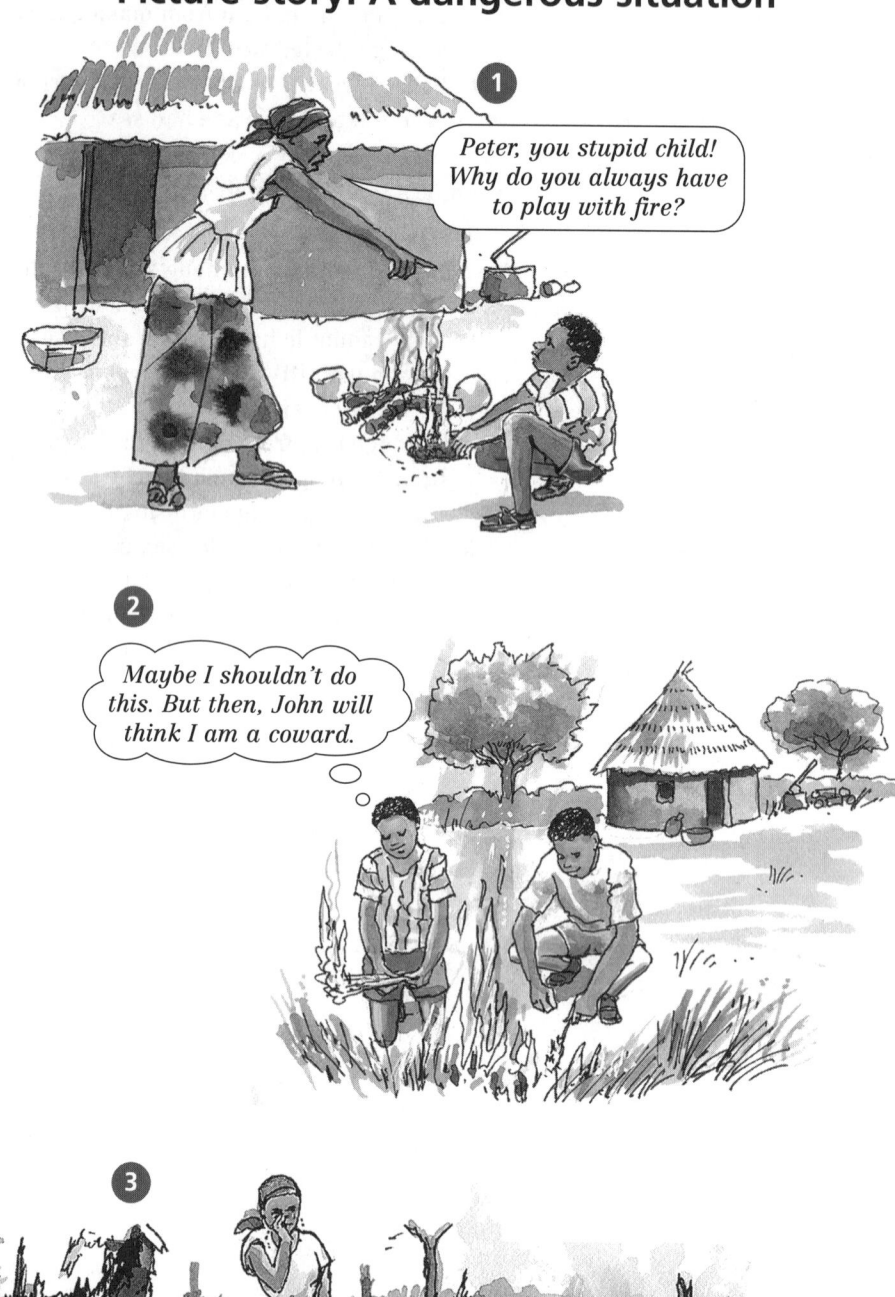

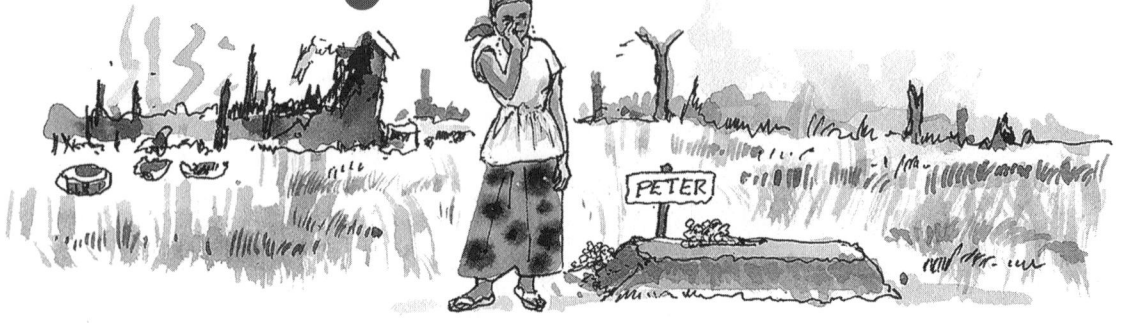

1 *Peter, you stupid child! Why do you always have to play with fire?*

2 *Maybe I shouldn't do this. But then, John will think I am a coward.*

3 PETER

*This picture also appears as part of Topic 22, page 46: **Changing the way we behave**.*

Teaching about HIV and AIDS

How young people's bodies develop

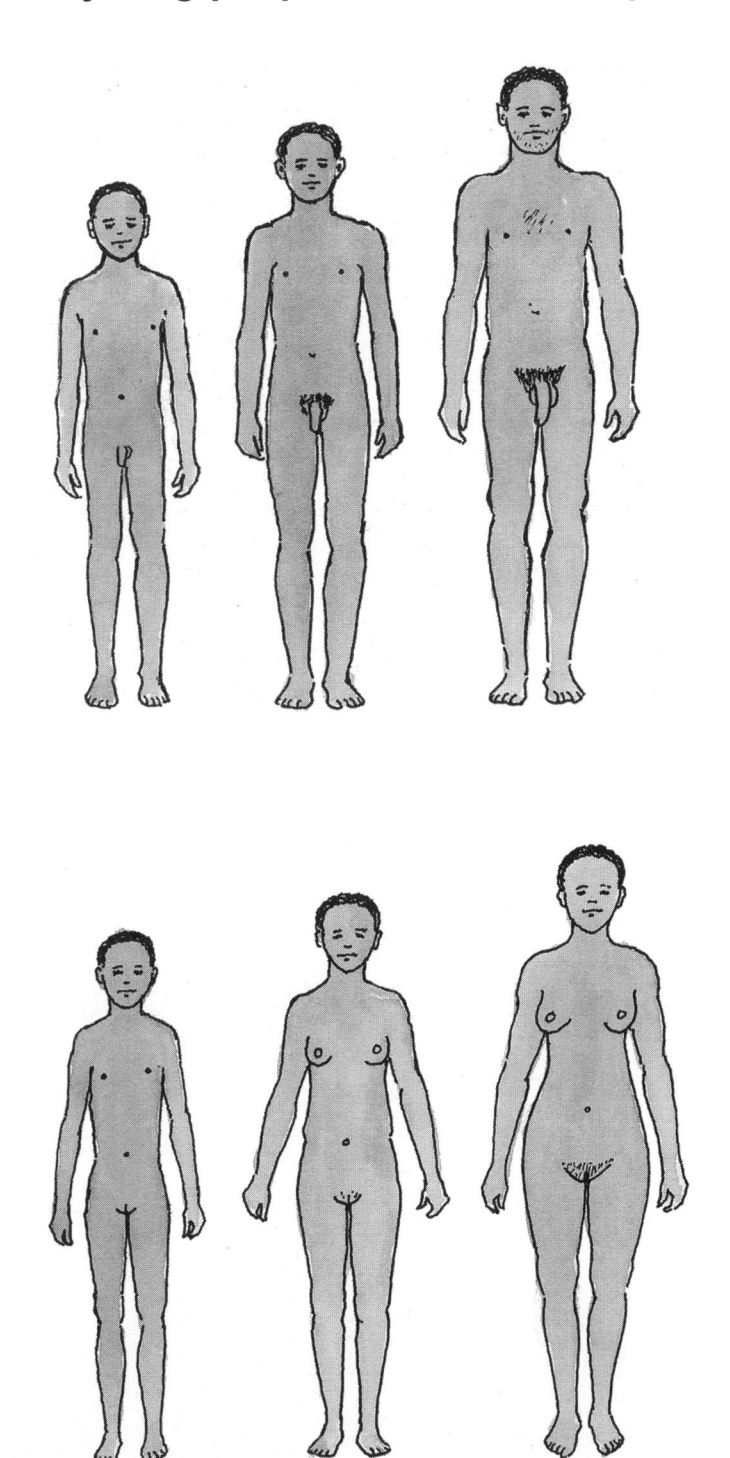

*This picture also appears as part of Topic 35, page 74: **Puberty: the changing body***